Inéo Hamed Ko

Initial breast cancer extension assessment using medical imaging

Inéo Hamed Ko

Initial breast cancer extension assessment using medical imaging

Multicenter study in Ouagadougou involving 502 cases

ScienciaScripts

Imprint
Any brand names and product names mentioned in this book are subject to trademark, brand or patent protection and are trademarks or registered trademarks of their respective holders. The use of brand names, product names, common names, trade names, product descriptions etc. even without a particular marking in this work is in no way to be construed to mean that such names may be regarded as unrestricted in respect of trademark and brand protection legislation and could thus be used by anyone.

Cover image: www.ingimage.com

This book is a translation from the original published under ISBN 978-620-6-72239-7.

Publisher:
Sciencia Scripts
is a trademark of
Dodo Books Indian Ocean Ltd. and OmniScriptum S.R.L publishing group

120 High Road, East Finchley, London, N2 9ED, United Kingdom
Str. Armeneasca 28/1, office 1, Chisinau MD-2012, Republic of Moldova, Europe
Printed at: see last page
ISBN: 978-620-8-18526-8

Contents

DEDICACES

I dedicate this work

A Peternel Dieu le pere tout puissant

I give thanks to ALLAH, the All-Merciful, the Most-Merciful, for everything he has blessed me with during my short life and my studies.

You are the king of glory, the one to whom nothing is impossible. I thank you for the privilege you have given me to study medicine and to carry out this work. Please bless my socio-professional career. May all the honour and glory be yours for centuries and centuries to come. AMEN!

To my mother Serme Djeneba

You are an inexhaustible source of tenderness, patience and sacrifice. Your prayers and blessings have been a great help to me along the way. Whatever I say or write, I cannot express enough my affection and gratitude to you. I hope never to let you down or betray your trust and sacrifices. You have never ceased to support and encourage me, and above all to pray for me throughout my years of study. On this memorable day for me and for you, please accept this work as a sign of my deep gratitude and my profound esteem. May the Almighty give you health, happiness and long life so that I can fulfil you in my turn.

To my father Ko Issoufou

Your endless patience, understanding and encouragement are the indispensable support that you have always given me. I owe you what I am today and what I will be tomorrow, and I will always do my best to remain your pride and never let you down. No words are adequate to express my deep feelings of love and respect; may the Almighty preserve you, grant you health, happiness and peace of mind and protect you from all harm.

To my twin brother Ko Inesseu Ь>таёl

Thank you for your encouragement and support. I wish you good health and a future full of joy, happiness and success in your life. Through this work, I express my feelings of brotherhood and love. May we always remain united.

To my brothers and sisters, KO Franck may your soul rest in peace, Abdoul, Aicha, IsmaSl, Bertrand and Christ

As a token of my brotherly affection, deep tenderness and gratitude, I wish you a life full of happiness and success. You are exceptional and I wish you every happiness. May Allah protect you, shower you with his graces and strengthen our brotherhood.

My Uncle Serme Yaya

You have spared no effort to accompany us whenever we needed it. Our prayer is that God will continue to shower you with his rich blessings.

To my uncle Dr Biyen Bely

We would like to express our sincere thanks for all your advice and support. May God continue to bless you and return your blessings a hundredfold. AMEN !!!

To My Uncle Number Seydou

Thank you for everything, may God continue to raise you beyond your expectations and may the best surprise you and your family.

ACKNOWLEDGEMENTS

Our thanks go to :

To my aunts and uncles

I won't mention any names for fear of forgetting some. Thank you to everyone for their many forms of support.

To my cousins

Thank you for your encouragement.

To my friends Zida, Sayouba, Cheick, Ibrahim, Ousmane, Prospere, Salimata

Thank you for being there every day and for supporting me. During these years of medicine, a distance may have been created with some of you, but I want you to know that I carry you in my heart. May God bless you abundantly and may he allow us always to share moments together.

To my friends from the promotion

Working alongside you has been one of the greatest legacies of my life. I have learnt from each and every one of you, and in your company I have become a better friend and future doctor.

May this mutual support continue throughout our lives as doctors and well beyond.

To Pr Ag. Benilde Marie Ange KAMBOU/ TIEMTORE my thesis supervisor

Thank you for agreeing to supervise this work. Thank you for your constant availability and encouragement, despite your very busy schedule. Over and above the professional side, you have provided us with support and maternal affection. Your humility and simplicity won us over. Your determination to get the best out of each and every one of your learners pushed them to excel. It was a great honour to learn from you, both in medical practice and in the legions of life. I pray to Almighty God to continue to inspire you with this great strength and to raise you to the pinnacle of your art. May he bless you and all your family.

To Dr Adjiratou KOAMA, my co-director

It is an immense honour for you to have co-directed this work. You have greatly contributed to its quality by guiding us, advising us and giving us a great deal of your precious time. We have been marked by your availability and your humility. We greatly appreciated your support and your valuable advice, which helped us to carry out this work. Your office was always open to us, with all the kindness and modesty that characterise you. In short, you are a role model for us. We hope that this work is acceptable, and the honour is all yours. Please accept the assurance of our esteem and sincere thanks. I feel fortunate to have

been with you for such a short time. May God bless you and your loved ones.
To all the staff in the medical imaging and interventional radiology department,
Thank you for your support and collaboration in producing this document.
To all breast cancer sufferers: Have faith in God and may He help you.
To bereaved families: May the Almighty be your comforter in this time of trial. Bless you.
To all those who have supported me in any way
I am also grateful to all the individuals and corporate bodies who, from near and far, have spared no effort to support the production of this document.

TO OUR ESTEEMED MASTERS AND JUDGES

To our master and president of the jury, Docteur Nayi Zongo (MCA)

You are :

> **Associate lecturer in surgical cancerology at the UFR SDS of the Joseph Ki Zerbo University,**

> **Oncology surgeon at CHUYO ,**

> **Former hospital intern in Burkina Faso**

> **Coordinator of the Master's degree in senology, cancer surgery techniques and breast reconstruction**

> **Coordinator of the National Cancer Control Programme (PNLCC)**

> **President of the Burkina Faso coalition against cancer (COBUCAN)**

> **President of the Burkina Faso League against Breast Cancer (LIBUCAS)**

> **Knight of the National Order of Merit of Burkina Faso**

Honourable Counsel :

It is a great honour for you to have agreed to chair this thesis jury, despite your many commitments. Your simplicity, your modesty, your constant availability, your rigour in your work and the breadth of your scientific knowledge make you an admirable man, a master appreciated by all. We had the privilege of benefiting from your theoretical and practical teaching during our training, during which we learned a great deal from you scientifically. Dear Master, allow us on this day to express our deep gratitude to you. May God guide you and bless you and your family; may he accompany you in all that you undertake. AMEN !

To our Honourable Master and Director of these Dr TIEMTORE-KAMBOU Benilde Marie-Ange (MCA)

You are :

> **Doctor, radiologist ;**

> **Associate lecturer in radiodiagnostics and medical imaging at the Unite de Formation et de Recherche en Sciences de la Sante (UFR/SDS) of the Joseph KI-ZERBO University;**

> **Head of the Medical Imaging and Interventional Radiology Department at the Bogodogo University Hospital;**

> **In charge of research, cooperation and innovation at the Societe Burkinabe de Radiologie (SOBURAD);**

> **Director of vocational training and national final examinations at the Ministry of Health and Public Hygiene;**

Dear Master,

Thank you for agreeing to supervise this work, thank you for your availability and your daily encouragement. Your love of a job well done, your demands on us to learn how to be a good doctor, your advice on a daily basis have helped to teach us rigour, discipline, the quest for excellence, but above all humility and respect for others. Beyond being a mentor, dear master, you have been a mother to us. You have guided us in the drafting of this document. Thank you is an understatement compared to the consideration you have shown us. We will always ask God to keep you and your family worthy of your kindness.

To our honourable master, Doctor Adjirata KOAMA épouse ZONGO, our thesis co-director

You are :

- **Radiologist at CHU-B ;**
- **Hospital practitioner at CHU-B ;**
- **Member of the Societe Burkinabe de Radiologie (SOBURAD), the Societe de Radiologie d'Afrique Noire Francophone (SRANF) and the Societe Frangaise de Radiologie (SFR);**
- **Member of the Ligue Burkinabe de lutte contre le cancer du sein (LIBUCAS).**

Dear Master,

Thank you for your availability and patience throughout this work, which has been a great research and learning experience for us. You spared no effort in giving us advice and encouraging us at every moment. You helped us to understand the full meaning of rigour and hard work. Your attention to detail has enhanced the quality of this document. I wish you a happy and fruitful career. May the Almighty bless you and your family beyond your expectations.

To our master and judge, Dr Ali P Ouedraogo

You are :

- **Maitre - assistant in radiodiagnostics and medical imaging at the Unite de Formation et de Recherche en Science De la Sante at the University of Ouayigouya;**
- **Radiologist at the Ouayigouya University Hospital;**
- **Deputy head of cooperation, research and innovation at the Société Burkinabe de Radiologie (SOBURAD);**
- **DFMS in radiodiagnostics and medical imaging at the Université Joseph Fourier Grenoble 2012;**
- **DIU d'imagerie de la pathologie osteo articulaire a Nancy en France 2012 ;**

> **DIU in senology at the Faculty of Medicine, University Lyon 1, France 2012**

Dear Master,

You are doing us a great honour by agreeing to judge this work despite your many requests. Your availability, your modesty and your sense of a job well done command our great respect. Please accept the expression of our deepest gratitude. May God bless you and shower you with his knowledge and wisdom in your career as a university hospitalist.

"By deliberation, the Unite de Formation et de Recherche en Science de la Sante, has decided that the opinions expressed in the essays to be presented are to be considered as the of their authors and that it and that it does not intend to give any approval or disapproval.

INTRODUCTION AND PROBLEM STATEMENT

Breast cancer is a malignant proliferation that develops in breast tissue [72,54]. It is a global public health problem because of its frequency and its morbidity and mortality. Breast cancer is the leading cancer worldwide, with 2,261,419 new cases expected in 2020 according to the World Health Organisation (WHO). One woman in 12 will be diagnosed with breast cancer in her lifetime [72,54]. It is estimated that around 685,000 women will die of breast cancer in 2020, making it the leading cause of cancer-related death in women worldwide [72,54]. In sub-Saharan Africa, breast cancer used to be the second most common cancer in women after cervical cancer [72,49], but according to the latest statistics from Global Cancer Statistics (GLOBOCAN), it is now the leading cause of cancer in many West African countries, including Burkina Faso.

Like other countries in sub-Saharan Africa, breast cancer is diagnosed late in Burkina Faso. Treatment is essentially medical and surgical. In recent months, the availability of radiotherapy has broadened the therapeutic arsenal. Imaging plays an important role at all stages of breast cancer management, for screening, extension assessment and follow-up [12]. Mammography is the first-line examination for the assessment of breast cancer [81]. MRI is used to assess the local spread of breast cancer, looking for multicentricity, multifocality and bilaterality [73]. Ultrasound of the axillary fossa is used to look for extension to the first lymph node. Thoracic-abdominal-pelvic CT and PET scans are used to investigate distant extension. Bone scintigraphy with MDP-Tc99m (SO) is commonly used in the assessment of extension and monitoring of breast cancer. However, authors are not unanimous about prescribing it as part of the initial staging of breast cancer, whatever its stage, and it has given rise to a number of articles. According to several authors, bone scintigraphy is justified in stages IIA to IV and not in stages 0 and I. The dorsal spine and costal gril are the most frequent sites of bone metastases at the stage of their discovery [24]. The initial extension work-up for breast cancer is not standardised; it depends on the stage of the tumour at the time of diagnosis, the warning signs, the teams involved and the technical resources available. In Burkina Faso, the inadequacy of the technical platform and the inaccessibility of the various examinations constitute an obstacle to health care in general and the initial breast cancer extension assessment in particular. PET scans are not available, and bone scans are not easily accessible, and can only be performed at the Yalgado Ouedraogo University Hospital (CHU-YO). The financial cost of these examinations is out of reach for the average citizen, especially as the guaranteed interprofessional minimum wage (SMIG) in Burkina, which comes into force on 1er July 2023, was set at 45,000 CFA francs, yet the average cost of a bone scan is 80,000 CFA francs and that of a thoraco abdominopelvic scan is 60,000 CFA francs. Despite these difficulties, breast cancer is routinely treated in Burkina Faso, and an initial extension assessment is always carried out. However, to the best of our knowledge, no study has yet been carried out on the initial extension assessment of breast cancer. The aim of this study was therefore to determine the different examinations prescribed in our context, and to identify the indications and factors associated with the prescription of different medical imaging examinations in the initial breast cancer work-up, in order to improve the management of breast cancer in Burkina Faso.

I PART

GENERAL

1. REMINDER

1.1.Embryology

> Mammary glands are modified apocrine glands of ectodermal origin that develop on either side of the body, along the mammary crete. During the 4^{e} week, an epidermal thickening, the mammary crete, appears on each side of the body. It extends between the roots of the limb buds. [62]

> More rarely, an ectopic nipple may be seen outside the mammary crete line, as a result of migration of the breast tissue.

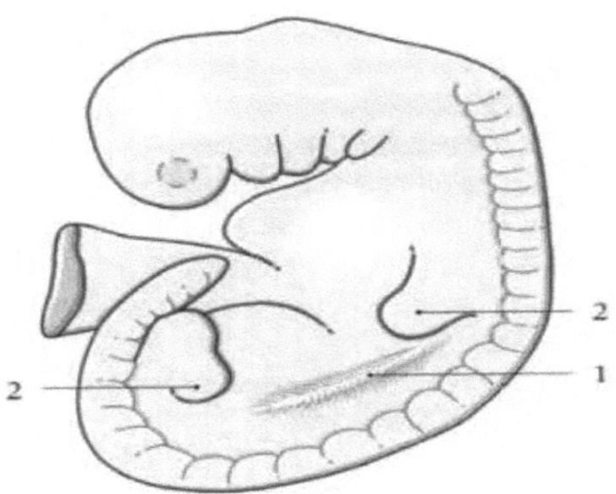

1.breast crete

2.draft members

Figure 1: Side view of a human embryo approximately 4 weeks old

During the 5^{e} week, the caudal part of the mammary crete disappears. The cranial part is reduced to a thickened epithelial mass, the primary mammary bud.

Rapid growth of the dorsal region leads to ventral transposition of the primary mammary buds. [62].

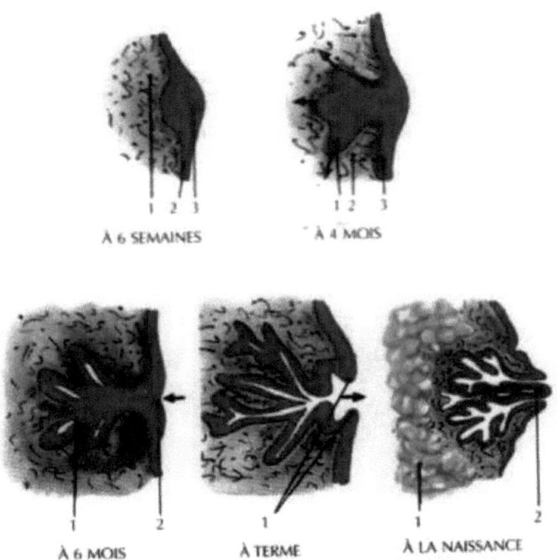

A6 WEEKS 1-mesenchyme 2-epiblast 3-mammary crete AT 4 MONTHS

1-mammary bud 2-derm 3-epidermis AT 6 MONTHS 1-canal galactophore 2-mammary fossa AT TERM 1-areola AT BIRTH 1-fat 2-mammary papilla

Figure 2: Organogenesis of the breast (cross-sections)

Between the 5th and 10th weeks, the appearance of the crete changes, its caudal part disappears and the cranial part is reduced to a thickened epithelial mass. This is the primary mammary bud [63].

Its rapid growth transforms it into several shapes; initially a disc, then a globe and finally a cone. From this point onwards, the nipple and areola are hollowed out [57].

From the 13th week, the deep surface of the mammary bud buds towards the underlying parenchyma, into which it sends solid cell cords; these are the embryos of the main galactophore ducts [44].

During the 15th week, differentiation of the lobular structure begins, starting with the galactophore ducts which develop a lumen and acquire their double cellular base: the cylindrical lining cells and the myoepithelial cells. These milk ducts open towards the nipple [44]. Thus, the fetus at term has a histologically complete and physiologically functional mammary gland [44].

1.2 Anatomical background

1.2.1. Definition

The breasts are paired glandular organs designed to secrete milk suitable for the nutrition of newborn babies, establishing intimate contact between mother and child. In addition to this main function, the breasts play a very important plastic (aesthetic) role in women, as well as an erogenous role due to their rich innervation [62].

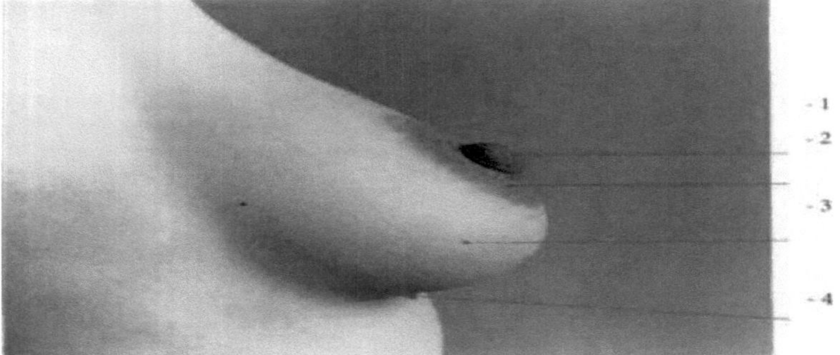

1 Nipple (mammary papilla**) 2** Areola
3. Peri-areolar skin **4.** Inframammary fold
Figure 3 : Female breast (side view)

1.2.2. Situation

The two breasts are located opposite the space between the 3eme and 7^e ribs. They are bounded by an inframammary fold and a supramammary fold, which is blurred, highlighted by the upward displacement of the breast.
This situation varies according to thoracic shape and type**.** [62].

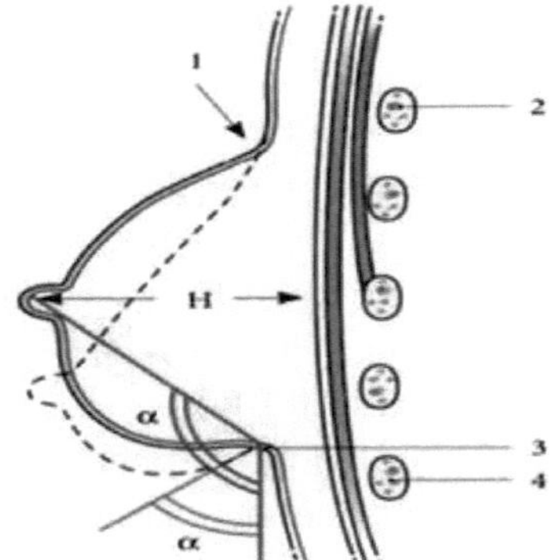

1. Supramammary fold
2. 3 e
3. Inframammary fold
4. 7 e

H. Nipple height
Figure 4: Parietal angle of the breast

1.2.3. Shape and dimensions

The general shape of the female breast is variable, most often conical and rounded. Insignificant before puberty; in young girls, the breasts have a semi-ovoid shape[62].

In adulthood, the breasts reach maturity, where their shape is roughly hemispherical to conical. Under the influence of its own weight (when standing) it tends to fall slightly[62].

With ageing, pregnancy and breastfeeding, the breasts will tend to ptosis and become more flaccid (more or less pendulous) [62].

In adults outside pregnancy, the breasts measure on average 10 to 11cm in height and 12 to 13cm in width[62].

Under the influence of pregnancy, the breasts increase in size shortly after implantation, but swelling often stops around the 4^e or 5^e month mark, only to resume at the end of gestation[62].

During breastfeeding, the breasts can double or even triple in size.

At the menopause, however, the volume of the gland gradually decreases[62].

1.2.4. Consistency - Weight

The breast is a skin gland with a slightly grainy consistency when palpated with a full hand, but this sensation disappears when pressed against the chest wall. It then appears firm and elastic. The average breast weighs 150g to 200g in young girls, and 400g or more in nursing mothers [62].

1.2.5. Reports and means of fixation

> **Reports :**

The breasts are connected to the skin at the front and to the musculo-facial and thoracic areas at the back.

> **Means of fixation :**

The main means of fixing the breast are the breast suspensory ligament and the skin.

1.2.6. External configuration

The skin covering of the breast is not homogeneous, and three zones are described:

> **Peripheral zone**: Smooth, supple and soft to the touch.

> **Middle zone:** this is the areola, pigmented and circular, 35 to 50 mm in diameter. Its appearance is made granular by voluminous sebaceous glands (MORGAGNI's tubercles). The glands become more

These are large during pregnancy and are known as MONTGOMERY tubercles.

> **Central zone:** this is the nipple; it occupies the centre of the areola and its pigmentation is identical to that of the areola. The milk ducts emerge through

orifices (2 to 20 orifices) [62].

1.2.7. Internal configuration

A sagittate section passing through the nipple shows from the surface downwards: the cutaneous envelope, the mammary body and the cellulo-fatty layer known as the retro-mammary layer [62].

Skin envelope: Three zones can be identified.

> **The peripheral zone:** the cellulo-fatty premammary tissue occupies this plane.

> **The middle areolar area:** the skin of the areola is thin and mobile, and is doubled by the areolar muscle (skin muscle).

> **The central zone or nipple:** its axis is occupied by the milk ducts surrounded by elastic connective fibres and smooth muscle fibres.

Mammary body or mammary gland: This is surrounded by a thin layer of connective tissue, the capsule. It is made up of several independent lobes [62].

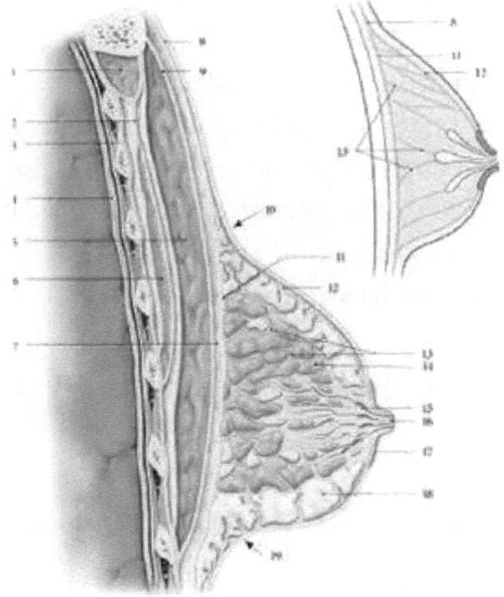

1 . m.subclavier
2 . fascia clavi pectoral
3 .endothoracic fascia
4 .pleve pariëtal
5 .m. pectoralis major
6 .m. pectoralis minor
7 .retro mammary space
8 .superficial thoracic fascia
9 .pectoral fascia
10 .supra mammary fold
Retro mammary fascia
12.premammary fascia

13.breast suspensory ligg
14.mammary lobule
15.lactiferous sinus
16.papilla 17.areole
18.premammary fat
19.inframammary fold

Figure 5: Sagittal section of the breast and chest wall

1.2.8. Vascularisation and innervation [62]

> Arterial vascularisation :

The internal part of the mammary gland is supplied by the perforating branches of the mammary gland, which pass through the first six intercostal spaces.

The external and inferior parts receive their blood from the external mammary artery, the inferior capsule of the superior acromiothoracic and thoracic arteries. One of these is more important than the others: this is the main external artery [62].

The mammary gland contains several branches of the intercostals. Most of the arteries approach the mammary gland from the superficial side. Retroglandular arteries are few in number[62].

> Venous vascularisation :

There is a superficial venous network, particularly visible during pregnancy and lactation, in which an anastomotic ring known as HALER's venous circle can sometimes be seen around the areola. This superficial network drains into neighbouring areas.

The deep veins drain into the external mammary veins to the outside, the internal mammary vein to the inside and the intercostal veins to the rear.

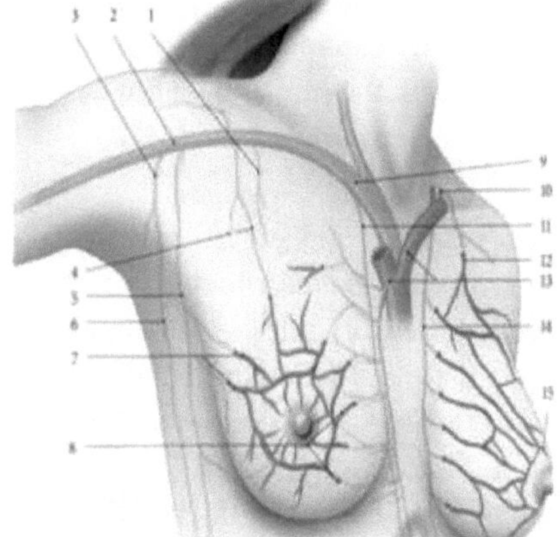

1. a. thoracic
2. a. axillary

3. a. subscapularis
4. Pectoral branch
5. a. lateral thoracic
6. a. thoracodorsal
7. Lateral mammary branch
8. Medial mammary branch
9. a. subclaviere
10. V. right jugular vein
11. a. internal thoracic
12. V. Mammary afferent
13. Brachiocephalic trunks
14. Internal thoracic vein
15. Periareolar venous ring

Figure 6: Arteries and veins in the breast

> Lymphatic channels :

Their importance in the dissemination of breast tumours is well known.

There are several chains, depending on where they are based:

- External mammary nodes: These arise below the lateral edge of the pectoralis major, in the middle of the axillary fossa, also following the course of the lateral thoracic artery.
- Internal mammary nodes: these follow the course of the internal mammary vessels within abundant fatty connective tissue. They are located above the endothoracic fascia in the intercostal spaces. The internal mammary lymphatic trunks drain into the thoracic duct on the left and into the lymphatic duct on the right.
- Crossed mammary gland lymphatics: The presence of nodes in the opposite breast to that affected by the carcinoma is probably simply the result of metastatic blockage of the usual lymphatic pathways and infiltration of the nodes of the opposite breast by retrograde route[62].

> Innervation :

A distinction is made between deep and superficial nerves:

- The deep nerves are sympathetic nets which travel to the gland via vessels.
- The superficial nerves are sensory nets which come from the supraclavicular branch of the cervical plexus, the thoracic branches of the brachial plexus, and the perforating branches of the 2nd, 3rd, 4th, 5th and 6th intercostal nerves.

All these nerves send numerous nets to the areola and nipple, which are therefore among the most sensitive areas of the body[62].

1.3.Physiological reminders

- **Action of gonadal hormones on the breast - ffistrogene :**

Astrogenes act directly on the excretory ducts of the mammary gland. Their action is sometimes direct, causing hyperhemia and sodium and water retention in the gland, as in premenstrual syndrome [57].

Astrogen stimulates the growth of the milk ducts, increases the mitotic index at the end of the duct and causes pigmentation of the areola. They stimulate the differentiation and development of the galactophorous epithelium.

- **Progesterone**

The direct action of progesterone on the mammary gland only seems to be possible if the gland has been previously prepared by astrogen.

It leads to alveolar-acinar proliferation, and complements the action of astrogenes to limit the growth of the galactophore ducts. It allows the acini to develop.

The indirect effect of progesterone seems to result from prolactin production. In the breast, progesterone counteracts the increase in capillary permeability caused by astrogens, and therefore reduces adematous phenomena **[57].**

The ovary is responsible for pubertal growth and maintenance of the gland during reproduction, with periodic modulation.

Total oophorectomy in young girls suppresses breast development at the time of puberty, but in adulthood there is little change in breast volume.

- **Action of extragonadal hormones - Prolactin :**

It is a pure protein hormone made up of a polypeptide chain of 205 to 211 amino acids. Prolactin acts on the acinus, causing secretion.

Its effector is the alveolar cell, where it leads to the synthesis of ribonucleic acid and lactose.

Excess prolactin reduces the cyclical function of the LH centre and inhibits the effects of gonadotropins on the ovary.

Prolactin acts in the mammary acini when it overcomes the peripheral inhibitor maintained by rnstrogens and progesterone **[44].**

- **Oxytocin :**

Oxytocin is secreted by the posthypophysis, which plays the role of alveolar emptying, and acts on a specific receptor, the myoepithelial cell of the mammary acinus, and the galactophoric ducts.

Non-innerve cells are sensitive to oxytocin and to mechanical stimulation, which explains why secretion is maintained.

Stimulation causes the alveoli to contract and the galactophores to dilate. It also promotes emptying of the acini.

- **FSH (follicle stimulating hormone) :**

It causes follicles to develop and astrogens (folliculin) to be secreted. It also develops and maintains secondary sexual characteristics**[44]**.

- **LH (luteinizing hormone):**

It causes ovulation with the formation of the corpus luteum and the secretion of progesterone.

- **The suprarenal gland and thyroid gland**

They appear to be involved in the development of mammary glands.

- **Physiological variations [44]**
- **The postnatal period:** the acini are the site of colostrogen secretion, which reaches its peak around 8^{e} days after birth. The breasts are tumefied and let out colostrum or "witch's milk".
- **The infantile period:** the galactophore ducts lengthen and the interlobular ducts branch out.
- **The pubertal period:** there is an increase in the connective stroma and a multiplication of the excretory ducts and acini, leading to an increase in the mammary body.
- **During the menstrual cycle:**

The first half of the cycle, under the effect of astrogen (proliferative phase), is marked by a multiplication of epithelial cells, a reduction in the lumen of the acini and an influx of lymphocytes into the connective tissue. The second half of the cycle, under the effect of progesterone (luteal phase), is characterised by dilation of the lumen of the acini, sometimes centred on intraluminal secretory material, a quiescent epithelium, vacuolation of the myoepithelial cells and a reddening of the connective tissue **[35,46].** These variations lead to a change in the volume of the breasts, which generally appear more tense, or even tender or painful.

- **During gestation:**

Pregnancy is accompanied by significant secretion of restrogCne and progesterone, together with placental lactogCne hormone and somatotropic chorionic hormone. During the first five months, the gland becomes congested, the capillary bed increases, the veins dilate, the lymphatics hypertrophy and there is a proliferation of ducts and acini. The last few months are marked by an accumulation of fat and basophilic granules at the apical pole of the acinar cells.

- **Lactation :**

After childbirth, the disappearance of the inhibitory effects of restrogCne and progesterone on prolactin induces lactation. The acini are distended by secretory material both in the cells and in the lumen of the lobular dactyloid units.

Once milk has been produced in the milk ducts, it is transported to the nipple via the milk ducts.

Milk production ceases within 7 to 10 days, if there is no stimulation by sucking on the nipple. However, it takes 3 to 4 months for the mammary parenchyma to return to its basal state **[15].**

During weaning, there is a regression of the acini and a reconstitution of fibroadipous tissue.

- **The menopausal period :**

The menopause is characterised by a progressive disappearance of the acini following a fall in estrogen and progesterone levels **[45].** Epithelial and myoepithelial cells atrophy and the basement membrane thickens. The connective tissue also changes, with alteration of the elastic fibres and collagen, leading to breast ptosis.

The breast of a menopausal woman is essentially made up of adipose tissue.

1.4.Histological background

1.4.1. Topographical histology

The mammary body is divided by connective tissue rich in adipose cells into several areas, which are known as lobes.

Each lobule is formed by a group of pedicle acini which join to form an interlobular duct. The union of several interlobular ducts forms a lactiferous duct, and all the lobules drained by a lactiferous duct form a lobe; there are around 15 to 20 per mammary body.

1.4.2. Structure [60]

> The acinus comprises a cavity bordered from inside to outside by :

> A layer of cubic cells with large chromatin-rich nuclei > A layer of myoepithelial cells (Boll basket cell); these are flat, star-shaped cells with small, dark nuclei and cytoplasm covered with myofibrils.

> A basal or vitreous membrane.

> The excretory ducts run from front to back:

> A vitreous which is gradually reinforced by an elastic conjunctival sheath **[60].**

> The myoepithelial cells that run the length of the ducts, a layer of cubic epithelial cells arranged in two layers at the level of the intra- and interlobular ducts, and in 3 or 4 layers at the level of the lactiferous ducts**[60].**

> The lumen of the lactiferous ducts is dilated to form a lactiferous sinus**[60].**

> The interstitial connective tissue is fairly dense in the interlobular region where the vessels and nerves travel, but becomes delicate in the lobules in contact with the alveoli, where the collagen fibrils are fine **[60].**

> The fundamental substance is abundant and there are many histiocytes: this is the alveolar "mantle", whose revolution also seems to be under hormonal control**[60].**

2. GENERAL INFORMATION ON BREAST DISEASES

2.1.Benign breast diseases

2012 WHO classification of breast lesions [80].

Benign breast disease is very common, occurring at all ages.

We have :

- **Benign epithelial proliferations**
- Adenosis sclerosante
- Apocrine adenosis
- Microglandular adenosis
- Radial scar/complex sclerosing lesion
- Breast adenofibroma
- Extraductal adenofibroma
- Lactating adenoma
- Adenosis sclerosante
- Fibrocystic mastopathy
- Fibroadenoma of the breast
- Atypical ductal hyperplasia
- Ductal ectasia
- Non-specific mastitis
- Mastitis subaigucus[1]
- Acute mastitis[1] , and chronic mastitis
- Fibrolipoma
- Fibrocystic dystrophy
- Epidermal cyst
- Cholesterolytic granuloma

2.2.Malignant breast diseases

- **Non-invasive carcinoma**
- **Lobular carcinoma in situ**
- **Invasive ductal carcinoma**
- Highly differentiated infiltrating ductal carcinomas, which include tubular and papillary infiltrating forms**[80].**
- Polymorphic carcinomas, which combine glandular areas and traveae.
- Atypical carcinomas have no glandular structure. They are made up of masses, trabeculae or isolated elements**[80].**
- Invasive lobular carcinoma
- Papillary carcinoma
- Cribriform carcinoma
- Mucosal carcinoma or colloid cancer
- Tubular carcinoma

- Spindle cell carcinomas

3. EPIDEMIOLOGY [60]

Breast cancer, which accounts for almost *12%* of all cancer cases worldwide, although its distribution is very uneven from one country to another and from one continent to another, as the following data shows, has become the most frequently diagnosed form of cancer in the world[60].

3.1.Geographical breakdown

Table I: Estimated increase (%) in the number of new cases and deaths from breast cancer, WHO Regions, 2020-2043

	WHO regions					
Estimated increase between 20202040 regardless of gender or age	**African Region**	**American Region**	**South East Asia Region**	**European region**	**Eastern Mediterranean Region**	**Western Pacific Region**
	%					
New cases of breast cancer	91,2	39,1	50,7	12,8	80,5	21,0
Deaths from breast cancer regardless of age	93,0	52,3	62,3	25,5	94,2	45,2

3.2.Etio-pathogeny : [3]

The etiology of breast cancer is not well known**[3]**. Cancer risk factors are often wrongly considered as factors that should play a role in the carcinogenic process. In reality, their only characteristic is a statistically significant link with the disease; their identification has a twofold interest**[3]** :

> To serve as a basis for the development of explanatory hypotheses to be verified by experimental studies;

> Identifying a subject who may be subject to increased surveillance: this is what should interest the practitioner.

3.3.The main contributing factors

> **Age**

The risk of developing breast cancer increases with age, even though it can affect women of different ages.

The risk of breast cancer in young women is low. Around 10% of cases of breast cancer occur in women under the age of 35, and almost 20% before the age of 50. Breast cancer most often develops around the age of 60. Almost 50% of breast cancers are diagnosed between the ages of 50 and 60, and around 28% are diagnosed after the age of 69.

> **History of breast cancer**

A woman who has had breast cancer is 3 to 4 times more likely to develop breast cancer again than a woman of the same age. This risk justifies regular and prolonged follow-up.

> **Breast disorders**

Among benign breast conditions, only those associated with the proliferation of breast tissue, such as hyperplasia, increase the risk of breast cancer. Women with atypical hyperplasia are 3 to 5 times more likely to develop breast cancer.

> **Exposure to medical radiation**

Chest irradiation can increase the risk of breast cancer. The level of risk is related to the total dose received and the woman's age.

Young women (before the age of 30) who have had repeated radiotherapy treatments of the chest or radiation treatment (radiotherapy) of the chest to treat another cancer (such as Hodgkin's lymphoma, for example) have a higher risk of breast cancer.

Women who have had a lung x-ray as a child (a type of x-ray that uses high doses of radiation) as part of the search for a primary tuberculosis infection (the body's first contact with the bacteria) have a higher risk of breast cancer.

> **Family background**

Almost 20% to 30% of breast cancers occur in women with a family history of cancer, including breast cancer, for example several cases of breast cancer in the same family.

> When a first-degree relative (mother, sister or daughter) has already had breast cancer, particularly if the diagnosis was made at a young age (before 50) before the menopause, the risk of developing this type of cancer is approximately twice as high;

> When second-degree relatives (such as a grandmother, aunt or niece on either side of the family) have already had breast cancer, the risk increases slightly.

> **Mutation of the BRCA1 and BRCA2 genes**

It is estimated that around 2 women in 1000 carry a BRCA1 or BRCA2 mutation.

These two genes are involved in repairing the damage that DNA undergoes on a regular basis. The presence of mutations in one of these two genes disrupts this function and greatly increases the risk of breast and ovarian cancer. However, not all women with these mutations will develop breast cancer one day.

Mutation of these genes increases the risk of developing :

> Breast cancer occurs at a young age, usually before the menopause. In a

woman carrying a BRCA1 or BRCA2 mutation, the risk of breast cancer varies from 40% to 80% over the course of her life, depending on the studies, the type of gene involved, the family history of breast cancer and her age;

> Cancer in both breasts (bilateral breast cancer) ;

> Ovarian cancer, mainly from the age of 40. The risk varies according to gene and family history.

> **Tobacco consumption**

Is associated with an increased risk of several cancers, including breast cancer. Recent studies have shown that women exposed to passive smoking (whose family and friends use tobacco) have a lower risk of breast cancer than those exposed to active smoking (who use tobacco themselves), but still higher than the risk of women never exposed to tobacco.

> **Alcohol consumption**

Is associated with an increased risk of several cancers, including breast cancer. It is thought to increase levels of restrogen, which itself plays an important role in the development of breast cancer cells.

The increased risk of breast cancer is significant from an average consumption of one glass a day. Reference studies attribute 17% of breast cancers to regular drinking, even moderate drinking.

> **Overweight/obesity**

Being overweight (BMI between 25 and 29.9) or obese (BMI of 30 or more) increases the risk of breast cancer in menopausal women.

3.4.Screening [3]

Breast screening makes it possible to detect any abnormality or cancer at an early stage, before any symptoms appear. This early detection increases the chances of recovery: 99 out of 100 women are still alive 5 years after diagnosis.

Screening for breast pathologies is based on :

> A mammogram (breast X-ray)

> A clinical breast examination (observation and palpation)

> Other examinations may be necessary, such as breast ultrasound, magnetic resonance imaging, breast cytology and histology. These additional examinations are common and do not necessarily mean that there is an abnormality. They can help the radiologist interpret the mammogram.

> **Palpation of the breasts**

Palpation of the breasts in the supine position, with the hands behind the head, explores the external and internal quadrants, the nipples and the sub- and retroareolar region of both breasts.

Palpation is performed using the pads of the three middle fingers, with three levels of pressure (superficial, intermediate and deep) for each small circular movement.

Its purpose is to look for the presence of a tumour or nodule:

> Painless, with a hard consistency or regular or irregular contours

> This may be associated with retraction or distortion of the nipple opposite, a skin fold, thickening of the areola with an orange peel appearance, and reddish, inflammatory skin.

3.5.Clinical and para-clinical studies

3.5.1. The clinic

3.5.1.1. Circumstances of discovery

The symptoms that lead patients to seek help vary. They may be :

> Pain: breast cancer is not usually painful, but you should be wary of persistent pain after your period.

> A tumour: this is the most common reason for the discovery of cancer

> A change in the skin or contour of the breast, or nipple discharge

> An abnormality of the nipple or areola, an isolated axillary adenopathy, a large arm

> A hematoma or spontaneous ecchymosis. The signs may be isolated or variously associated.

3.5.1.2. Questioning

It states:

> The date and conditions in which the lesion appeared,

> Whether or not it is painless,

> Any changes in volume,

> Pregnancy and breast-feeding,

> Current hormone treatments,

> Medical and surgical history,

> Risk factors.

3.5.2. Physical examination

> **Inspection**

With good lighting, from the front, from the side, then with a sloping daylight. She is looking for :

- Wrinkles, folds, redness, an orange peel appearance or depression of the skin during mobilisation;
- A change in subcutaneous circulation;
- On the nipple: retraction, spontaneous discharge, a raspberry-eczematiform appearance;
- An erythemato-ulcerous erosion with a yellowish crust on the nipple may

suggest Paget's disease.

> **Palpation**

- **Palpation of the mammary gland**

Fingers are laid flat, quadrant by quadrant, including the nipple area, the para-mammary area and the axillary extension. It shows the consistency of the glands and whether or not they are homogeneous. If a nodule is palpated, its nature is determined:

- Firm or hard
- Regulated or not
- Good or bad limits.

Its greatest diameter is measured, and its precise location in the breast is noted on a dated diagram. We will also look for adhesion.

- On the skin: depression caused by mobilisation of the tumour or the surrounding skin;
- Nipple: attracted or deformed when the tumour is mobilised or the tumour is mobilised when the nipple is mobilised;
- To the pectoralis major: by contracting it with a counter-clockwise adduction.
- (Thillaux's manoeuvre). The tumour does not normally follow the movements of the muscle, unless it is adherent to it;
- In the chest wall: the tumour is deeply fixed, even when the muscle is relaxed.

We also look for nipple discharge caused by pressure on the nipple or one of the quadrants of the breast.

> **Palpation of the axillary and supra-clavicular hollows**

- It scrapes the ribcage medially, and the examiner insinuates his fingers towards the top of the axillary fossa, behind the tendon of the pectoralis major muscle, then finishes on the outside.
- We will be looking for one or more adenopathies, the nature of which we will specify (common; hard and irregular (suspicious), mobile or attached to each other or to other parts of the axillary fossa).

The clinical examination will be thorough, examining the liver, spleen, lungs and heart for any metastases.

3.6. Paraclinical examinations

3.6.1. Diagnostic check-up

> **Mammography**

Mammography is a radiological examination dedicated to the study of the breast. It is carried out using an X-ray machine dedicated solely to this purpose: the mammograph. Mammography can be carried out either as part of a breast cancer screening programme (screening mammography), or in the presence of symptoms (diagnostic mammography) [38]. Mammography cannot tell whether a lesion is liquid or solid. Breast density alters the sensitivity of analogue mammography and leads to more false positives. The superinternal part of the breast and the retro areolar region are difficult to analyse on frontal and external oblique views.

> **BI-RADS classification of lesions [31].**

A classification called BI-RADS (Breast Imaging Reporting and Data System) from the American College of Radiology (ACR) classifies the images described into seven (7) diagnostic evaluation categories. Each category corresponds to a certain degree of probability of having breast cancer. On the basis of a rigorous radiological semiology, this classification will appear in the conclusion of the reports (CR) in order to determine the course of action (CAT) and specific follow-up methods if necessary. BI-RADS classification (Breast Imaging Reporting and data System) of the American College of Radiology ACR**[31].**

ACR 0: This is a wait-and-see classification that is used in screening situations or while waiting for a second opinion, before the second opinion is obtained or the imaging work-up is complete and allows a definitive classification to be made. Additional investigations are necessary: comparison with previous documents, additional incidences, central views, compressed views, enlargement of microcalcifications, ultrasound.

ACR 1 no abnormalities: mammogram normal.

ACR 2 Round opacities with microcalcifications :

- Intramammary ganglion
- Round opacity corresponding to typical cyst(s) on ultrasound Image(s) of fatty or mixed density
- Known scar(s) and calcification(s) on suture material
- Microcalcifications without opacities, There are benign abnormalities that do not require monitoring or further examination.
- Annular or arciform, semi-lunar, sedimented, rhombohedral microcalcifications
- Cutaneous calcifications and diffuse regular punctiform calcifications.
- ACR 3: A solid mass with regular contours and no calcification.

Focal asymmetry of density, isolated grouping of punctiform microcalcifications. This is probably a benign anomaly (-2% risk of malignancy) requiring close monitoring.

- ACR 4: ACR4A: PPV of cancer between 2 and 10%.

Partially circumscribed mass corresponding on ultrasound to a solid nodule suggestive of a fibroadenoma, an isolated cyst with complications or a probable

abscess. ACR4B: PPV of cancer between 10 and 50%.
Grouping of fine polymorphous or amorphous microcalcifications, a solid mass with indistinct contours.
ACR4C: PPV of cancer between 50 and 95%. Newly appeared solid mass with indistinct contours, new focus of fine linear microcalcifications. There is an indeterminate or suspicious abnormality, which indicates that histological verification is required.
ACR 5 Arboreal vermicular microcalcifications or irregular, polymorphic or granular microcalcifications, numerous and grouped Grouping (clusters) of microcalcifications whatever their morphology, whose topography is galactophoric. Microcalcifications associated with an architectural anomaly or opacity. Grouped microcalcifications which have increased in number or microcalcification whose morphology and distribution have become more suspect. Poorly circumscribed opacities with blurred and irregular outlines. Spiculated opacities with dense centres. There is an abnormality suggestive of cancer. The lesion must be biopsied to obtain a diagnosis **[31]**.
ACR 6: Proven cancer. Surgery must be performed if clinically indicated.

- **Breast ultrasound**

A proven and effective diagnostic imaging technique, breast ultrasound uses high-frequency ultrasound waves for imaging, Doppler evaluation and elastography [51]. Breast ultrasound is the most important complementary examination after mammography [37]. This examination completes and clarifies the images obtained by mammography. It does not replace mammography, which is the reference examination for the breast.

- **Taking the test**

The examination is carried out in the supine position, with the arm raised and the side to be analysed slightly elevated, quadrant by quadrant, in orthogonal planes, not forgetting the submammary fold, the parasternal regions, the axillary areas and the retro areolar region. It is always bilateral, comparative and accompanied by careful palpation [37].

- **Indications [51]**

Breast ultrasound is used in particular for the following indications:

- Examination of abnormalities detected by palpation and skin changes;
- Examination of serous or bloody nipple discharge;
- Examination for persistent, non-cyclical pain or tenderness in a specific area of the breast;
- In-depth evaluation of ambiguous or abnormal mammographic results;
- The first imaging technique to be used for the assessment of clinical abnormalities in women aged under 30 and in pregnant or breast-feeding

women;

- MRI-guided ultrasound (second look) ;
- Assessment of problems associated with breast implants;
- Planning treatment with postoperative curietherapy ;
- Screening of high-risk patients who are unable or unwilling to undergo MRI screening;
- Guidance for intervention ;
- Axillary lymph node assessment and biopsy for staging of ipsilateral breast lesions that are (or are likely to be) malignant;
- Follow-up of probably benign lesions (type 3 according to the BIRADS method) detected by ultrasound, such as possible fibroadenomas and complex cysts.

Breast ultrasound is not indicated for :

- General population screening,
- Ongoing monitoring of confirmed single cysts.

3.6.2. Extension assessment

- **Locoregional extension [65]**

Axillary ultrasound if not performed. The currently recommended indications for breast MRI (HAS) are :

- in cases of high risk of multifocal or multicentricity (lobular cancer)
- if the conventional balance sheet is in danger of failing
- in the event of a difficult therapeutic choice (before oncoplastic surgery, before neoadjuvant chemotherapy, etc.).

- **Axillary ultrasound**

This is an imaging technique that uses ultrasound to visualise the axillary fossa. It is able to detect major lymph node involvement based on morphological abnormalities such as cortical thickening, peripheral vascularisation, hilar infiltration and loss of the lymph node's reniform appearance. Axillary exploration is essential, as it assesses the regional extent of the disease, making it one of the major prognostic factors. Various pre-operative imaging examinations may reveal involvement of these axillary lymph nodes. However, the reference imaging remains axillary ultrasound, which can also be used to guide sampling. The role of imaging is even more important. The aim of ultrasound is to avoid a two-stage curage after a positive sentinel node.

- **Magnetic resonance imaging (MRI) [65].**

MRI (Magnetic Resonance Imaging) of the breast does not replace mammography or breast ultrasound. It is not a systematic examination for the diagnosis of breast cancer. It is an additional tool. Bilateral breast MRI will be proposed if**[65]** :

- Age < 40
- Known or 1st degree BRCA mutation, high family risk (Eisinger score) - Neoadjuvant treatment programme: recommended
- Suspicion of multiple cancers on standard imaging, and if conservative surgery is being considered
- Discrepancy in tumour evaluation (> 10 mm) between the clinic and standard imaging or between mammography and echo, with an impact on the surgical procedure.
- Surgery with programmed oncoplasty
- Invasive lobular cancer (option, not recommended by HAS) to be discussed on a case-by-case basis (no proven benefit)
- On a case-by-case basis in other clinical contexts, such as extremely dense breasts

Angiomammography can be an alternative to MRI

The data published show :

- Sensitivity equivalent to MRI for index cancer
- Slightly (but not significantly) lower sensitivity of angiomammography compared with MRI for additional cancers,
- Significantly better specificity of angiomammography/MRI (less risk of false positive results)
- False negatives on MRI are mainly CLI and CCIS (but often with visible Ca+).

> Assessment of distant extension [65].

There is no systematic recommendation**[65].** Clinical clues or pejorative prognostic factors should be taken into account**[65]**. **In** view of the low prevalence observed in patients with invasive T1 and T2 tumours without clinical lymph node involvement, it is not recommended to carry out a systematic extension work-up in the absence of clinical clues in these patients**[65].** In practice, extension imaging is recommended for cT3-T4 or cN+ tumours (whether or not patients receive neoadjuvant systemic treatment); however, the value of extension imaging in T1 N1 tumours seems questionable after surgery, in the case of macrometastatic lymph node invasion**[65].** The first-line work-up may be based on one of the following three options:

- Chest X-ray, abdominal ultrasound and bone scan;
- or thoracoabdominal CT scan and bone scan;
- or 18 F-FDG PET-CT**[65].**
- **Bone scintigraphy [17]**

Bone scintigraphy is a nuclear medicine test used to analyse the function of all bones and joints. The principle is to use a slightly radioactive product used for bone function. The product used for this type of examination will bind to the bones and joints, enabling all bone and joint pathologies to be identified. Advantages of bone scintigraphy: - Allows all visible lesions to be detected 2 to 12 months before the X-ray.

- It explores the whole body.
- She has great sensitivity.
- Recommendations concerning bone scintigraphy [23] ;
- A baseline bone scan for all patients in stages II to IV, regardless of tumour size.
- All tumours larger than 2 cm, because there is a risk of metastases even if patients are asymptomatic, because 32% of patients with metastases are asymptomatic.

- **Chest X-ray**

Radiography is based on the use of X-rays. The beam is emitted from a fixed, non-rotating source (a tube). The rays are absorbed more by the tissues, depending on their density, before being collected by a photosensitive film placed behind the patient. The X-rays leave a more or less opaque trace on the film, depending on the density of the tissue they pass through. Chest X-rays are used to analyse differences in lung density. The presence of multiple opacities with more or less homogeneous water density, rounded shapes, clear boundaries and regular contours in the lung fields, giving a balloon-like appearance, is indicative of pulmonary metastases. However, many authors find that CT is more sensitive and reliable for pulmonary metastatic lesions.

- **18 FDG PET scan**

Positron emission tomography (PET) is a quantitative and dynamic functional imaging technique developed in nuclear medicine departments and in experimental settings. The general principle of PET imaging is based on the use of radio tracers labelled with a positron-emitting isotope (beta plus radiation) and dedicated cameras. The images obtained provide a non-invasive, in vivo, three-dimensional representation of the volume distribution of the radioactive signal within the body. In this way, the volume concentration of radioactivity and the tissue kinetics of the radiotracer can be monitored over time. PET imaging requires relatively extensive logistics and the involvement of many different professions. FDG PET is recommended:

- If recidivism is suspected
- Staging a known recurrence
- High risk of recurrence; young people under 40, triple negative, HER2

positive, lymph node involvement, residual disease after neoadjuvant treatment

- For clinically superior stage II B breast tumours, preferably before surgery.
- In the case of prevalent axillary lymph node metastases (search for other metastatic sites)
- FDG PET is not recommended for the extension assessment of clinically stage I breast tumours.
- Invasive breast cancer T3, T4 or N plus
- Before neoadjuvant chemo
- Triple negative cancer, HER2 overexpressed or amplified, T2N OR Pn1Mi

❖ **Abdominal ultrasound**

The ultrasound image is formed by the reflection of ultrasound waves emitted by the transducer from the tissues. The reflected waves are picked up by the transducer and processed electronically, so the ultrasound images obtained are projected onto the screen. Ultrasound reflection depends on the impedance of the tissue. The echo texture of normal liver is considered as normal echo gene. Hepatic metastases are the most common malignancy of the liver. In the case of metastases, the changes in the hepatic echo structure are: hyperechogenic nodules in 60% of cases, multiple giving a snowstorm image; hypoechogenic nodules in 20% of cases, multiple giving a colander image, cocarde nodule with hypoechogenic centre and hyperechogenic periphery. The number of nodules varies. Ultrasound provides an objective view of the shape and echo structure of the liver, although CT is better at characterising hepatic nodules.

❖ **TDM Thoraco abdomino pelvic**

A scanner is a medical imaging technique that involves measuring the absorption of X-rays by the patient's tissues and reconstructing two- or three-dimensional images of the human body. An external source of X-rays irradiates the patient, and these are detected by a detector located on the other side of the patient. The source and detector rotate around the patient. The X-rays generated in the X-ray tube pass through the patient's body, interacting to a greater or lesser extent with the tissues.

A thoracic-abdominal-pelvic CT scan is used to study the thorax, abdomen and pelvis, as well as the vascular network and the skeleton from the thoracic vertebrae to the pelvis. TAP is a widely used examination in the assessment of breast cancer extension.

II PART

OUR STUDY

1. OBJECTIVES

1.1.General objective

Study of the initial extension assessment of breast cancer in Ouagadougou.

1.2.Specific objectives

1. To determine the sociodemographic characteristics of patients who have undergone an initial breast cancer extension assessment;
2. To study the clinical characteristics of patients who have benefited from the initial breast cancer extension assessment;
3. To describe the diagnostic imaging and histological aspects of breast cancer in our study;
4. Identifying the imaging examinations performed in the initial breast cancer work-up in Ouagadougou;
5. To compare the imaging examinations carried out in the initial extension assessment of breast cancer in Ouagadougou with international standards;
6. To determine the factors associated with the prescription of different medical imaging examinations in the initial work-up for breast cancer;

2. METHODOLOGY

2.1.Scope of the study

Our study took place in the medical imaging, obstetric gynecology and oncology departments of hospitals in the city of Ouagadougou in Burkina Faso, in particular the Bogodogo University Hospital (CHU-B), the YALGADO OUEDRAOGO University Hospital (CHU-YO) and the SCHIPHRA Protestant Hospital.

2.1.1. YALGADO OUEDRAOGO University Hospital Centre (CIU YO)

Created in 1958 and in operation since 1961, the CHU-YO is a reference hospital in Burkina Faso. Located in the city of Ouagadougou, CHU-YO comprises the Department of Medicine and Medical Specialities, and the Department of Surgery and Surgical Specialities. As a national reference centre, it offers specialised care to patients in the peripheral structures referred to it, and is involved in the diagnosis, medical and surgical management of breast cancer.

2.1.2. Bogodogo University Hospital Centre (CIU-B)

It is one of the 3rd level hospitals in the healthcare system, having absorbed the former Centre medical avec antene chirurgicale (CMA) in sector 30, and is located in sector 51 of the city of Ouagadougou. It is spread over two sites, namely the site of the former CMA in sector 30 (known as site B) and the newly-built site (known as site A). The organisation of care at CHU_B is based around medical and technical services. It provides care for cancer patients, particularly breast cancer patients, and houses the country's first radiotherapy centre.

2.1.3. Schiphra Protestant Hospital

The Schiphra Protestant Hospital was founded in Ouagadougou in 1953 by the missionary Pierre Dupret and his wife. The Schiphra Protestant Hospital is a hospital with medical and technical services. It provides medical, surgical and follow-up care for patients suffering from breast cancer.

2.2.Sampling method

Sampling was exhaustive, including all available reports of initial breast cancer extension examinations performed during the study period.

2.3.Sample size

Calculation of the sample size using the Schwartz formula :

$n = z^2 \times p\ (1 - p) / m^2$;

n=sample size ;

z = 95% confidence level, z = 1.96, for a 99% confidence level, z = 2.575);

p = proportion when unknown, p = 0.5 is used;

m = margin of error tolerated 5% pres ;

N = population size ;

N/(N+n) = correction coefficient ;
With a confidence level of 95% and a margin of error of 5%;
n = (1.96) 2 x (0.5) (1-0.5) / (0.05) 2 = 383 ;
Our minimum sample size should be 383 patients according to the Schwartz formula. To increase the statistical power of our sample, we decided to take a minimum of 400 patients.

2.4.Data sources

The reports were compiled from the archiving system for reports from medical imaging departments, clinical records of patients in the gynaecology and medical and surgical oncology departments, and general surgery departments of the Bogodogo and Yalgado teaching hospitals and the Schiphra Protestant Hospital.

2.5.Inclusion criteria

Reports from breast cancer patients who underwent an initial extension work-up during the study period in hospitals in the city of Ouagadougou were included.

2.6.Exclusion criteria

Incomplete or unusable extension work-up reports for breast cancer patients were not included. Examinations carried out as part of the follow-up assessment.

2.7.Type and period of study

This was a descriptive-analytical study covering a 3-year period from 1er January 2021 to 31 December 2023, with retrospective data collection.

2.8.Variables studied

The following variables were taken into account in our study:

- **Socio-demographic data**: age, gender, place of residence, level of education and occupation;
- **Antecedents;**
- **Clinical data ;**
- **Paraclinical data ;**
- **Therapeutic data ;**

The variables were collated using an individual data collection form and the Kobocollecte electronic data collection system.

2.9.Operational definitions

Initial extension work-up: this is a series of tests designed to determine the stage at which the cancer has progressed and whether it has spread to other organs in the form of metastases. The aim of the initial extension assessment is to determine the most appropriate treatment. It is the first imaging test carried out immediately after confirmation of the diagnosis.

2.10. Data analysis

The data collected was entered and processed on a microcomputer using EPI

Info software in its French version 7.2.2.6; the figures were produced using EXCEL 2016 and WORD 2016.

2.11. Ethical and deontological considerations

The study protocol was submitted to the institutional ethics and medical deontology committee of Bogodogo University Hospital. Authorisation for the study was requested and obtained from the Directors General of each hospital; the confidentiality of the information collected was strictly respected, as was anonymity.

3. RESULTS

Flow chart showing the total number of patients and the number of patients per university hospital and hospital.

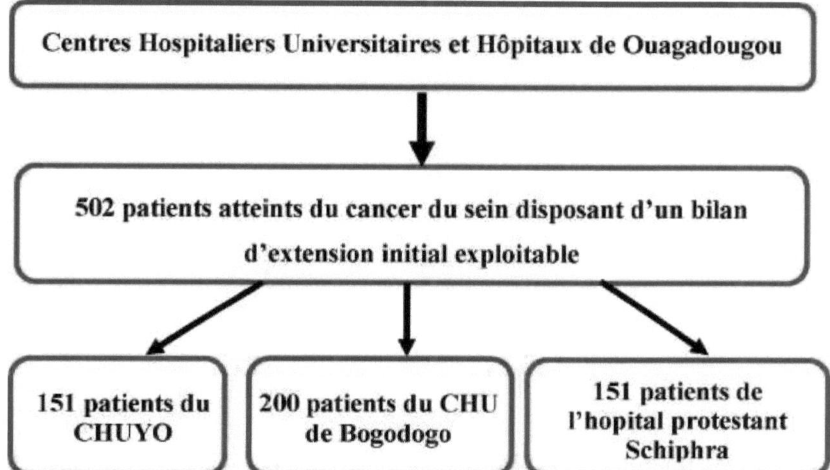

Figure 7: Flow chart showing the distribution of our study population by university hospital and hospital

3.1.Socio-demographic characteristics

3.1.1. Age

The mean age of our patients was 48.53 ±12.29 years, with extremes of 19 and 86 years. The 40-50 age group was the most common, representing 32.87% of all patients. The distribution of patients by age group is shown in Figure 1.

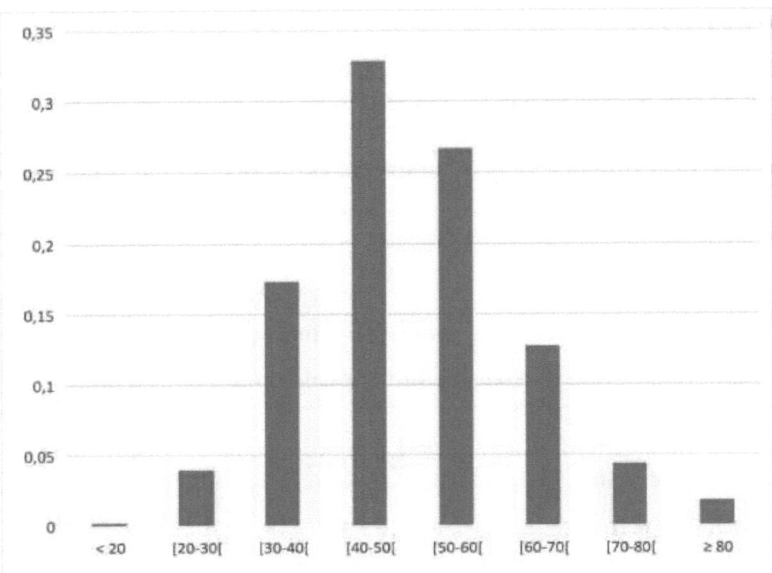

Figure 8 : Distribution of patients having undergone the initial breast cancer extension assessment, by age group (N= 502)

3.1.2. Gender

Women represented 98.41% (494 cases) of the population compared with 1.59% (8 cases) of men.

3.1.3. Source

Patients came from urban areas in 72.71% of cases (365 cases), compared with 27.29% (137 cases) from rural areas.

3.1.4. Level of education

Primary school patients were the most represented, accounting for 38.65% of cases, while those with no formal education accounted for 30.68% (154 cases).

Table II: Distribution of patients having undergone the initial breast cancer extension assessment according to level of education (N=502 cases).

Level of education	Workforce	%
Primary	194	38,65
No level	154	30,68
Secondary and university	154	30,68
Total	**502**	**100,00**

3.1.5. Socio-professional category

Housewives represented the majority of our population with 60.76% of cases, or 305 patients.

Table III: Breakdown of patients who underwent initial breast cancer extension assessment by socio-professional category (N=502 cases).

PROFESSION	Workforce	%
Housewife	305	60,76
Employee	112	22,31
Commergant	35	6,97
Cultivator	21	4,18
Other professions	21	4,18
Contractor	8	1,59
Total	**502**	**100,00**

3.2.Clinical characteristics

3.2.1. History of gynaecological cancer and oral contraception

A family history of breast cancer was found in 4.38% (22 cases) of patients and ovarian cancer in 0.80% (4 cases). Oral contraception was used in 23.11% of patients (116 cases). The distribution of patients according to antecedents is shown in Table IV.

Table IV: Breakdown of patients who underwent the initial breast cancer extension assessment according to previous history of gynaecological cancer and oral contraception

History of oral contraception and gynaecological cancer	Workforce	%
History of oral contraception	116	23,11
Family history of breast cancer	22	4,38
Personal history of breast cancer	19	3,78
Family history of ovarian cancer	7	1,39
Personal history of ovarian cancer	4	0,80

ATCD : antecedents

3.2.2. Management and parity

The majority of our patients were multigestate and multiparous. Tables V and VI show the distribution of patients according to gestation and parity respectively.

Table V: Distribution of patients according to gestite (n = 494)

Obstetrical history Gestite	Number (n=494)	%
Nulligest	22	4,58
Primigeste (1 pregnancy)	50	10,16
Paucigeste (2-3 pregnancies)	143	28,49
Multiple gestation (4-5 pregnancies)	141	28,88

Large multiple gestation (> 5 pregnancies)	138	27,89
Total	**494**	**100**

Table VI: Distribution of patients according to parity

Obstetric history Parite	Number (n=494)	%
nulliparous	34	6,97
Primipare	54	10,96
Paucipare	148	29,88
Multipare	144	29,08
Large multiparous	114	23,11
Total	**49 4**	**100**

3.2.3. Menarches

The age of menarche was 14 in the majority of our patients, and 33% of our patients had their menarche after the age of 14.

Table VII: Breakdown of patients by age of menarche

Age of the menarches	Number (n=487)	%
11	3	0,62
12	40	8,21
13	109	22,38
14	172	35,32
15	110	22,59
> 16	53	10,88
Total	**487**	**100,00**

3.2.4. Circumstances of discovery

The most common reason for discovery was a nodule or breast mass in 99% of cases. The breast was inflammatory in 49.4% of cases. Table VIII shows the distribution of patients according to the circumstances of discovery.

Table VIII ^ Distribution of *patients* according to circumstances of discovery

Circumstances of discovery	Number (n=502)	%
Breast lump or nodule	497	99,00
Inflammatory breast	248	49,40
Axillary adenopathy	84	16,73
Breast ulceration	21	4,01
Abnormal breast discharge	15	2,99
Pruritus	6	1,20
Tingling	4	0,80
Asymmetrical breasts	2	0,40

Lymphredeme	2	0,40
Breast pain	1	0,20
Breast induration	1	0,20
Umbilical nipple	1	0,20
Breast retraction	1	0,20
Breast tension	1	0,20
Cough	1	0,20

3.2.5. General condition

The majority of patients were in good general condition, with 69.72% in WHO stage I. Table IX shows the distribution of patients according to general condition.

Table IX : Distribution of patients having undergone initial breast cancer work-up according to general condition

Stage (WHO)	Number (n=502)	%
I	350	69,72
II	79	15,74
III	55	10,96
IV	18	3,59
Total	**502**	**100,00**

3.2.6. Location of the tumour

The left breast was the most common site, accounting for 48.21% of patients.

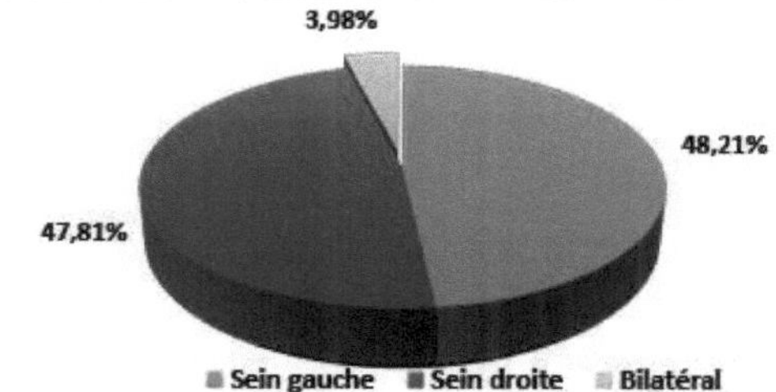

■ Left breast Right breast ■Bilateral

Figure 9: Distribution of patients having undergone initial extension work-up according to tumour location

3.2.7. Clinical signs found

Breast nodules, inflammatory breast and adenopathy were the most common clinical signs.

Table X : Distribution of patients who underwent initial breast cancer work-up according to clinical signs found

Clinical signs	Number (n=502)	%

Breast lump or nodule	501	99,80
Inflammatory breast	457	91,04
Axillary adenopathy	346	68,92
Respiratory sign	46	9,16
Spinal pain	13	2,59
Neurological sign	17	3,39
Abdominal sign	19	3,78
Breast ulceration	25	4,98
Breast discharge	10	1,99
Lymphredeme	4	0,80
Asthenia	1	0,20
Big, heavy arms	1	0,20
Umbilical nipple	1	0,20
Retracted skin	1	0,20
Linear breast wound	1	0,20
Presence of vegetation	1	0,20
Bleeding	1	0,20
Menstrual disorders	1	0,20

3.3 Paraclinical characteristics

3.3.1. Histological type

Non-specific infiltrating carcinoma (CINOS) represented 90.84% (456 cases) of histological types.

Table XI: Distribution of patients having undergone initial breast cancer work-up according to histological type

Histological type	**Number (n=502)**	**%**
Non-specific invasive carcinoma	456	90,84
Invasive lobular carcinoma	15	2,99
Mucinous carcinoma	9	1,79
Invasive squamous cell carcinoma	4	0,80
Phyllodes carcinoma	4	0,80
Sarcoma	3	0,60
Adenocarcinoma	2	0,40
Metaplastic carcinoma	2	0,40
Atypical hyperplasia	2	0,40
Intra-ductal papilloma	2	0,40
Invasive carcinoma	1	0,20
Medullary carcinoma	1	0,20
Tubular carcinoma	1	0,20
Isolated hyperchromatic cells	1	0,20

3.3.2. Histopronostic grade

Scarff Bloom and Richardson grade 2 modified (mSBR) by Elston and Ellis represented 69.32% (348 cases) of cases.

The distribution of patients according to cytological grade is shown in Figure 14.

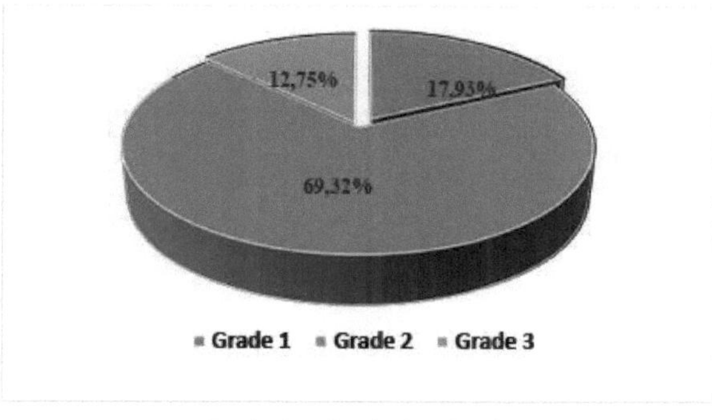

Grade 1 Grade 2 Grade 3

Figure 10: Distribution of patients according to histopronostic grade mSBR

3.3.3. Presence of vascular emboli

Vascular emboli were present in 63 cases (12.55%) compared with 439 cases (87.45%).

3.3.4. Diagnostic imaging

Table XII : Distribution of patients having undergone initial breast cancer work-up according to diagnostic imaging work-up

Imaging	Number (n=502)	%
Echo Mammography	236	47,01
Breast ultrasound	203	40,44
Mammography	106	21,12
No	5	1

3.3.5. Brest Imaging and Data System (BIRADS) classification from the American College of Radiology (ACR)

The majority of lesions were classified as ACR 4 and ACR 5.

Table XIII: Distribution of patients who underwent initial breast cancer work-up according to ACR lesion classification

ACR	Number (n=502)	%
ACR3	27	5,38
ACR4	204	40,64

ACR5	271	53,98	
Total	**502**		**100,00**

3.3.6. Imaging examinations in the initial extension work-up

A thoracic-abdominopelvic CT scan was the most commonly performed examination, involving 77.29% of patients.

Table XIV: Distribution of patients having undergone the initial breast cancer extension work-up according to the actual imaging test performed

Imaging tests	Number (n=502)	%
CT-thoraco-abdomino-pelvic	388	77,29
Abdominal ultrasound	277	55,18
Chest X-ray	256	51,00
Chest scan	43	8,57
Bone scan	16	3,19
Axillary ultrasound	11	2,19
Breast MRI	9	1,79
Abdominal and pelvic CT scan	7	1,39
Thoracic angioscan	5	1,00
Radiography of the spine	2	0,40
Echo Doppler	1	0,20
Cerebral scanner	18	3,59
Cerebral MRI	2	0,40

Abdominal ultrasound, chest X-ray and thoracic-abdominal-pelvic CT scan were the most frequently performed examinations at stage 2.

Table XV: Distribution of patients having undergone the initial breast cancer extension work-up according to the examinations carried out at stage 2

Imaging tests	**Stage 2 patients**	
	Number (n=68)	%
Thoracic-abdominal-pelvic scan Abdominal ultrasound Chest X-ray Chest CT scan Axillary ultrasound Breast MRI	45 4667 ,65 4566 ,18 11,47 11,47 11,47	66,18

A thoracic-abdominopelvic CT scan was the most frequently performed examination at stage 3 (70.37%).

Table XVI: Breakdown of patients according to examinations carried out at stage 3

Imaging tests	Stage 3 patient Number (n=243)	%
Thoracic-abdominal CT scan pelvic	171	70,37
Abdominal ultrasound	141	58,02
Chest X-ray	135	55,56
Chest scan	14	5,76
Bone scan	3	1,23
Axillary ultrasound	10	4,12
Breast MRI	4	1,65
Abdominal and pelvic CT scan	4	1,65
Cerebral scanner	2	0,82

The thoracic-abdominopelvic CT scan was the examination the realest in stage 4, i.e. 89.01% of patients.

Table XVII: Distribution of patients having undergone the initial extension work-up according to the examinations carried out at stage 4

Imaging tests	Stage 4 patients Number (n=191)	%
Thoraco-abdomino-pelvic scanner	170	89,01
Abdominal ultrasound	90	47,12
Chest X-ray	75	39,27
Chest scan	27	14,14
Bone scan	13	6,81
Breast MRI	4	2,09
Abdominal and pelvic CT scan	3	1,57
Thoracic angioscan	1	1,00
Radiography of the spine	2	0,40
Cerebral scanner	16	8,38
Cerebral MRI	2	1,05

3.3.7. Local extension

Nipple involvement was the most frequent local extension.

Table XVIII : Distribution of patients having undergone initial breast cancer work-up according to local extension

Local extension	Number (n=502)	%
Skin damage	275	54,78
Damage to the nipple	95	18,92

Multifocal tumour	58	11,55
Multicentric tumour	49	9,76
Bilateral tumour	20	3,98

3.3.7. Metastases

The thorax was the most common site of metastasis with 49.27%. Nodules were present in 84.44% of cases, and pleural tumours in 25.93%.

Table XIX: Breakdown of patients who underwent initial breast cancer work-up according to the location of metastases

Metastasis	**Number (n=274)**	**%**
- Thoracic metastasis	135	49,27
Lung nodule	114	84,44
More than 3 pulmonary nodules	74	54,81
Pulmonary micronodules	10	7,41
Less than 3 pulmonary nodules	9	6,67
Pleuresie	35	25,93
- Metastases abdomino-pelvic	66	24,09
Hepatic metastases	62	93,94
More than 3 liver nodules	51	77,27
Less than 3 liver nodules	6	9,09
- Bone metastases	57	20,80
Spinal location	45	78,95
Basin location	15	26,32
Dimensional locations	18	31,58
Other locations	6	10,53
Cerebral metastases	16	5,84
Total	**274**	**100,00**

3.3.8. TNM classification

Table XX: Breakdown of patients who underwent the initial extension work-up of the
breast cancer according to TNM classification

Tumour	**Number (n=502)**	**%**
T2	75	14,94
T3	145	28,88
T4	282	56,18
Total	**502**	**100,00**
Ganglion	**(n=502)**	**%**
N0	4	0,80
N1	282	56,18

N2	206		41,04
N3		10	1,99
Total	**502**		100,00
Metastasis		**(n=502)**	**%**
M0	312		62,15
M1	191		37,85
Total	**502**		100,00

3.3.9. Stage

Table XXI: Breakdown of patients who underwent initial extension work-up of breast cancer by stage according to TNM classification

Stadium	Number (n=502)	%		%
Stage 2	**68**	**13,55**		
T2	N0	M0	2	2,94
T2	N1	M0	58	85,29
T2	N1	M1	1	1,47
T2	N2	M0	4	5,88
T3	N0	M0	2	2,94
T3	N1	M0	1	1,47
Stage 3	**243**	**48,41**		
T2	N1	M0	3	1,23
T2	N2	M0	1	0,41
T2	N3	M0	2	0,82
T3	N1	M0	80	32,92
T3	N2	M0	26	10,70
T4	N0	M0	1	0,41
T4	N1	M0	65	26,75
T4	N2	M0	65	26,75
Stage 4	**191**	**38,05**		
T2	N1	M1	72	37,70
T2	N2	M1	107	56,02
T2	N3	M1	8	4,19
T4	N2	M0	4	2,09

Table XXII: Breakdown of patients who underwent initial extension work-up

breast cancer by stage

	Number (n=502)	%
Stage 2	68	13,40
Stage 3	243	48,40
Stage 4	191	38,20

Total	502	100,00

Table XXIII: Breakdown of patients having undergone initial breast cancer work-up according to treatment

Treatment	Workforce	%
Chemotherapy	423	84,26
Mastectomy	363	72,31
Axillary Curage	357	71,31
Radiotherapy	14	2,79
Conservative surgery breast	5	1,00
Hormonotherapy	3	0,60

3.3.10. Bi-varied analysis

> Relationship between thoracic-abdominal-pelvic CT and socio-demographic characteristics, stage and management of patients

There was a statistically significant association between the level of secondary or university education, salaried occupation and the performance of a thoracoabdominopelvic CT scan. Thoracoabdominopelvic scanning was associated with secondary and university education with a P.value of 0.9%, and salaried occupation and business occupation were associated with thoracoabdominopelvic scanning with P.values of 0.2% and 0.00% respectively. There was no statistically significant association between place of residence and thoracoabdominopelvic scanning.

Table XXIV: Correlation between thoracic-abdominal-pelvic CT scan and socio-demographic characteristics of breast cancer patients undergoing initial extension work-up

Variables	OR (IC :95%)	P-value
Residence		
Rural	1,42[0,90-2,23]	0,06
Urban	1	
Level of education		
Primary	0,75[0,49-1,15]	0,09
Secondary and university	1,77[1,08-2,89]	**0,009**
No level	0,81[0,51-1,26]	0,17
Profession		
Employee	2,20[1,12-3,96]	**0,002**
Housewife	1,06[0,69-1,62]	0,39
Contractor	2,07[0,25-17,05]	0,27
Cultivator	0,93[0,33-2,61]	0,43

Commergant	0,27[0,13-0,55]	**0,00**

There was a statistically significant association between thoracic and abdominopelvic CT scans and TNM stages. Stages 3 and 4 were associated with the performance of a thoracoabdominopelvic CT scan during the initial extension work-up with a P. value of 0.02. This association was positive with an oder ratio of 1.73, i.e. stage 3 and 4 patients were 1.73 times more likely to have a thoracoabdominopelvic CT scan during the initial extension work-up than stage 2 patients.

There was a statistically significant association between thoracoabdominopelvic CT scan and chemotherapy. Chemotherapy was associated with the performance of a thoracoabdominopelvic CT scan during the initial extension work-up, with a P. value of 0.00. This association was positive: patients undergoing chemotherapy were 3.23 times more likely to have had a thoracoabdominopelvic CT scan during their initial breast cancer extension work-up.

Table XXIIII: correlation between thoraco-abdominopelvic CT scan and treatment during initial breast cancer work-up

Variables	OR (IC :95%)	P-value
Surgery		
Yes	0,76[0,47-1,24]	0,13
No	1	
Chemotherapy		
Yes	3,23[1,95-5,38]	**0,00**
No	1	

> Relationship between chest radiography and socio-demographic characteristics, stage and management of patients undergoing initial breast cancer work-up

There was a statistically significant association between level of education, occupation and the performance of chest radiography during the initial breast cancer work-up. The absence of educational level was associated with the performance of thoracic radiography with a P.value of 0.004; the occupation of shopkeeper was associated with the performance of thoracic radiography during the initial breast cancer work-up with a P.value of 0.006. These associations were positive with respective order ratios of 1.66 and 2.55.

Table XXIVI Correlation between chest radiography and socio-demographic characteristics during the initial breast cancer work-up

Variables	OR (IC :95%)	P-value
Residence		

Rural	1,31[0,88-1,95]	0,08
Urban	1	
Level of education		
Primary	0,81[0,57-1,17]	0,13
Secondary and university	0,75[0,51-1,10]	0,07
No level	1,66[1,13-2,44]	**0,004**
Profession		
Employee	0,82[0,54-1,26]	0,19
Housewife	0,88[0,62-1,27]	0,25
Contractor	0,31[0,06-1,57]	0,07
Cultivator	1,29[0,53-3,13]	0,28
Commergant	2,55[1,19-5,43]	**0,006**

There was a stastistically significant association between the TNM stage of the breast cancer and the performance of a chest X-ray during the initial extension work-up. Stages 3 and 4 were associated with the performance of a chest X-ray with a p.value of 0.002.

Table XXVI: correlation between chest radiography and TNM stage in the initial breast cancer work-up

Variables	OR (CI:95%)	P-value
Stadiums		
TNM classification		
Stages 3 and 4	0,47[0,27-0,80]	**0,002**
Stage 2	1	

There was a statistically significant association between chest radiography and chemotherapy during the initial breast cancer work-up with a P value of 0.008. This association was negative with an order ratio of 0.05.

Table XXVIX: correlation between the performance of chest radiography and the management of patients with breast cancer during the initial extension work-up.

Variables	OR (IC :95%)	P-value
Surgery		
Yes	1,12[0,75-1,65]	0,28
No	1	
Chemotherapy		
Yes	0,05[0,33-0,9]	**0,008**
No	1	

> **Relationship between the performance of abdominopelvic ultrasound,**

socio-demographic characteristics, stage and patient management

There was a statistically significant association between the performance of abdominopelvic ultrasound and the level of secondary and university education, and the absence of level at the time of the initial breast cancer work-up with a P value of 0.01 and 0.005 respectively. There was also a statistically significant association between the performance of abdominopelvic ultrasound and commercial occupation with a P.value of 0.00.

Table XXVII: Correlation between the performance of abdominopelvic ultrasound and socio-demographic characteristics during the initial breast cancer work-up.

Variables	OR (IC :95%)	P-value
Residence		
Rural	0,88[0,59-1,31]	0,26
Urban	1	
Level of education		
Primary	0,93[0,65-1,33]	0,35
Secondary and university	0,66[0,45-0,96]	**0,01**
No level	1,65[1,11-2,44]	**0,005**
Profession		
Employee	0,63[0,41-0,96]	0,01
Housewife	1,02[0,71-1,46]	0,44
Contractor	0,8[0,20-3,27]	0,38
Cultivator	1,08[0,44-2,62]	0,43
Commergant	3,5[1,49-8,17]	**0,00**

There was a statistically significant association between abdominopelvic ultrasound and TNM stage 3 and 4 in the initial breast cancer work-up with a P value of 0.01.

There was a statistically significant association between the performance of abdominopelvic ultrasound and chemotherapy treatment during the initial breast cancer work-up with a P value of 0.001.

Table XXVIIII: correlation between abdominopelvic ultrasound and treatment

Variables	OR (IC :95%)	P-value
Surgery		
Yes	1,16[0,78-1,71]	0,23
No	1	
Chemotherapy		
Yes	0,44[0,26-0,75]	**0,001**
No	1	

> **Relationship between bone scintigraphy, socio-demographic characteristics, stage and patient management**

There was a statistically significant association between the performance of a bone scan and rural residence at the time of the initial breast cancer work-up, with a P value of 0.002.

Table XXIXI: Correlation between bone scintigraphy and socio-demographic characteristics during the initial breast cancer work-up

Variables	OR (CI:95%)	P-value
Residence		
Rural	Nd	**0,002**
Urban	1	
Level of education		
Primary	1,05[0,37-2,94]	0,47
Secondary and university	0,42[0,15-1,16]	0,05
No level	1,18[0,71-14,19]	0,05
Profession		
Employee	2,15[0,76-6,05]	0,08
Housewife	0,63[0,23-1,72]	0,19
Contractor	0.00[Nd-Nd]	0,38
Cultivator	0.00[Nd-Nd]	0,49
Commergant	0,50[0,11-2,33]	0,20

There was no statistically significant association between bone scintigraphy and TNM stage in the initial breast cancer work-up.

There was no statistically significant association between the performance of a bone scan and treatment during the initial breast cancer work-up.

Table XXX: correlation between the performance of bone scans and CEP

Variables	OR (IC :95%)	P-value
Surgery		
Yes	1,15[0,36-3,64]	0,42
No	1	
Chemotherapy		
Yes	2,86[0,37-22,02]	0,15
No	1	

> **Relationship between brain scans, socio-demographic characteristics, stage and patient management**

There was a statistically significant association between the performance of brain scans and rural residence and the level of secondary and university education at the time of the initial breast cancer work-up, with a P. value of 0.01 and 0.04 respectively.

Table XXXII: correlation between brain scan and socio-demographic characteristics during the initial breast cancer work-up

Variables	OR (CI:95%)	P-value
Residence		
Rural	6,65[0,86-50,04]	**0,01**
Urban	1	
Level of education		
Primary	1,01[0,38-2,65]	0,48
Secondary and university	2,33[0,90-6,01]	**0,04**
No level	1,45[0,99-3,71]	0,32
Profession		
Employee	1,78[0,65-4,86]	0,13
Housewife	0,63[0,24-1,62]	0,1
Contractor	0.00[Nd-Nd]	0,74
Cultivator	0.00[Nd-Nd]	0,45
Commergant	0,77[0,1-6,02]	0,45

There was a statistically significant association between cerebral CT and TNM stage 3 and 4 in the initial breast cancer work-up with a P. value of 0.03.

There was a statistically significant association between the performance of brain scans and chemotherapy during the initial breast cancer work-up, with a P. value of 0.02.

Association of patients having undergone the initial breast cancer extension work-up between thoracoabdomiopelvic scanner + scintigraphy =16 patients

Association of patients who underwent initial breast cancer work-up between abdominopelvic ultrasound + chest X-ray + bone scan = 0 patients

4. DISCUSSION

4.1.Limits of the study

Our study had a number of limitations in its implementation. The quality of the data was affected by the retrospective nature of the study, and by incomplete completion and poor maintenance of medical records. Despite these objective limitations, we obtained results that we have discussed and commented on in the light of the literature.

4.2.Age

The mean age of the patients in our study was 48.53 years, with extremes ranging from 19 to 86 years. The most common age group was 40 to 50 years. Our data are close to those of Sidibe in Mali (47.44%) [66] and those of Kiendrebeogo et al [41] and Bambara et al [9] in Burkina Faso. This average age is higher than that of Sinnadurai [67] in China (in 2019) and Umoke et al [77] in Nigeria (in 2019), which were 39.47 and 42.9 years respectively. Breast cancer is diagnosed most frequently at around 63 years of age in France according to Dabakuyo-Yonli [20] (in 2020), and at 63.4 years of age in the United States according to Kirkpatricket al. [42] in (2021). Certain studies suggest the existence of a racial and ethnic disparity in the age of diagnosis of breast cancer in women [78,79]. Women of colour are more likely to develop breast cancer at a younger age than their white counterparts [34,70]. This is thought to be due to a disparity in exposure to risk factors, and largely to underlying social and economic inequalities [29], which are very marked between developing and industrialised countries [64].

The relatively young age of onset of breast cancer in our study could be explained by the youth of the Burkinabe population; and the fact that women at this age (perimenopause) have already been exposed to certain cancer risk factors such as oral contraception, excess weight and sedentariness [64].

The health of Burkina Faso's population is influenced by lifestyle behaviours and climate change [52,53]. In addition, African women living in urban areas are likely to lose the protective benefits of low exposure to estrogen, as their parity decreases, their first pregnancy occurs at a later age and they reach menopause [49].

4.3.Background

In the present study, a family history of breast cancer was found in 4.38% of patients. This rate is lower than those of Anwar et al [5] in Indonesia (in 2019) and Bakkach et al [8] in Morocco (in 2017), which were 15% and 22% respectively. Breast cancer is characterised by certain genetic alterations (especially mutations in the BRCA 1 and 2 genes) which are hereditary and can be transmitted from generation to generation [18,50]. This makes a family history of breast cancer an important risk factor for breast cancer [6]. Prevention of breast cancer would be improved by searching the general population for people with a family history of breast cancer, using a large-scale survey, looking for genetic abnormalities in this group. The aim is to identify them and to monitor these individuals through screening and special periodic follow-up.

4.4.Clinical and histological features

In the study, the left breast predominated with 48.21%. Our results were similar to those of Bambara et al [9] , Delma in Burkina Faso [21] and Engbang et al [26] who found the same thing with 51.25%, 55% and 52% respectively. In our study, tumour involvement was unilateral in 96.02% of cases. This result is close to those of Umoke et al [77] in Nigeria (in 2019) and Bakkach et al [8] in Morocco (in 2017) in whom tumour involvement was mostly unilateral with respective rates of 87.3% and 100%. The unilateral nature was due to infiltrating carcinomas of the nonspecific type, which represented the majority of the tumours.

90,84 % [2,16]. This characteristic could influence patient survival, in the sense that studies suggest that unilateral cancers have a better prognosis than bilateral cancers which are associated with a gene mutation or a more aggressive cancer [36,82].

4.5.Histological type

Non-specific infiltrating carcinoma was the most common histological type with 90.84%. Our results are similar to those of Bambara (93.75%) [9], Guindo in Mali [30], Soudre (86.96%) in Burkina Faso [69], Anwar et al. [5] in Indonesia (in 2019), Umoke et al. [77] in Nigeria (in 2019) and Aka et al [1] in Cote d'Ivoire (in 2021), the majority of whom reported non-specific infiltrating carcinoma, with rates of 80%, 76.4% and 90.4% respectively. Kirkpatrick et al [42] in the United States (in 2021) also reported infiltrating carcinoma in 93.2% of cases. Non-specific infiltrating carcinoma is the most common histological type of breast cancer [33]. It represents an advanced form of tumour disease compared with carcinoma in situ. The high proportion of invasive carcinomas in our study could be explained by the non-adherence of certain women at risk to systematic breast cancer screening, for several reasons. Many women are still diagnosed at an early stage [11,19]. This may be due to socio-cultural factors that foster prejudice, a lack of information about breast cancer, and a therapeutic itinerary that begins with recourse to traditional medicine [76]. However, diagnostic facilities are only available in hospitals, and usually in urban centres. This could constitute an obstacle to early detection. A low level of education, lack of awareness of breast cancer, poor knowledge of early diagnosis methods, financial constraints and limited access to healthcare are possible reasons for

this delay in diagnosis [27].
In the study T3/T4 predominated with 85.06%, this is comparable to that of Some in Burkina Faso which found 77% [68] and that of Kemfang in Cameroon which found 77.25% [40]. However, it is higher than the Maydouline series in Casablanca (26.41%) [28]. The therapeutic itinerary of patients is strongly affected by socio-cultural beliefs underpinned by a low level of education in our populations. Ignorance of the curability of breast cancer, which is still associated with death, the stigmatisation of cancer patients, and the non-practice of breast self-examination are all factors contributing to the long consultation times frequently reported in sub-Saharan Africa [22,49,56,76]. This would explain the predominance of stage T3/T4 tumours with lymph node involvement, or even metastatic disease, at the time of diagnosis, as seen in our African context [7].

4.6.Histopronostic grade

Scarff Bloom and Richardson grade 2 modified (mSBR) by Elston and Ellis was the most frequent histopronostic grade with a rate of 69.32%. Our result is close to that of Bakkach et al [8] in Morocco (in 2017) who reported a grade 2 mSBR with a rate of 47.6%. However, our result differs from that of Anwar et al [5] in Indonesia (in 2019) who found that the majority of mSBRs were grade 3 with a rate of 78.5%. Intermediate grade 2 remains in the majority of reported studies [8]. The mSBR grades give an idea of the degree of aggressiveness of the tumour. It represents an obligatory histopronostic factor reported on pathological anatomy reports. The SBRm II grade found in the study is linked to the fact that non-specific infiltrating carcinoma was the most frequent histological type found, with a rate of 90.84%. In addition to being the most frequent, non-specific infiltrating carcinoma is an aggressive tumour. Its aggressiveness is linked to a high frequency of indifferent cancers (grades II and III) and greater tumour insensitivity to hormones (absence of astrogen receptors) [19].

4.7.Therapeutic aspects

4.7.1. Surgery

In our study, 72.2% underwent surgery. Surgery was radical in the majority of cases. It was a mastectomy associated with lymph node dissection in 71.12% of cases. Our results are comparable to those of Anwar et al [5] in Indonesia (in 2019) in whom radical surgery (mastectomy plus axillary curage) was performed in 84% of cases. Our results could be explained by the fact that the majority of women were already close to the menopause and no longer had much interest in keeping the affected breast. In fact, age is associated with the choice of type of surgery. Younger women remain attached to changes in their body image because of the demands of married life. They have a greater demand for conservative surgery than older patients. We also found that tumour size was associated with the type of surgery. Conservative surgery focuses on tumours that are less than or equal to 3 cm in size, with a low tumour/breast volume ratio. The development of senology could make it possible to offer better care, combining improved survival and quality of life. Axillary dissection was associated with radical surgery. The advanced stages at diagnosis, with axillary lymph node invasion, justified its routine practice in our context. Sentinel lymph node surgery requires a rather special technical platform. However, it would reduce the complications associated with lymph node dissection, which would have fewer indications [83].

4.7.2. Radiotherapy

Radiotherapy reduced the absolute risk of locoregional recurrence by 15.7% and the absolute risk of death by 3.8% [48]. However, only 14 patients benefited from this treatment. This low rate in our study is due to the fact that Burkina Faso did not inaugurate its first radiotherapy centre until 2021 [22]. Prior to this, patients were obliged to travel outside our borders to countries with better technical facilities for radiotherapy treatment. This option, which increased the cost of treatment, was out of reach for most patients.

4.7.3. Chemotherapy

In our series, 84.26% received neoadjuvant and adjuvant chemotherapy. The most commonly used protocols were AC60, FAC and taxane. This rate is close to those of Anwar et al [5] in Indonesia (in 2019) and Bakkach et al [8] in Morocco (in 2017), which were 68.6% and 61.7% respectively.

4.8.Diagnostic imaging

Mammography and breast ultrasound are the gold standard for the early detection of breast cancer. They are the diagnostic tool that has reduced breast cancer mortality in the West [55,65]. Unfortunately in our context, systematic screening remains a national project and individual screening is the preserve of women with financial means and education. Apart from the 5 cases of necrotic ulcerated lesions which did not require a diagnostic work-up, diagnostic imaging was performed in 99% of cases in our series. According to the classification of the American Society of Radiology (ACR), which is widely used by radiologists, biopsy is required as soon as the mass is classified as BIRADS 4 or above [13;32;55;61:65;]. Masses classified as BIRADS 3 are said to be potentially benign, but require radiological surveillance, with no immediate obligation to request a biopsy [4, 55]. For BIRADS 4 and 5 lesions, the malignancy rate is over 70% [13, 61]. In our study, 93.62% of cancers diagnosed were classified as BIRADS 4 or 5 on imaging. This testifies to the ability of medical imaging to detect the vast majority of cancerous lesions [39].

However, tumours initially classified as BIRADS 3 (5.38%), biopsied either because of their clinical appearance or the patient's history, turned out to be genuine breast cancers. In the Burkinabe context, these discrepancies are thought to be due to inadequate mastery of the BIRADS classification or to African specificities, which suggest that a higher number of cancers appear benign on radiology [55]. Several factors may account for the interpretation errors reported in the literature [10,14,59,61]. In 42% of cases, these errors are due to errors of perception, in 15% to errors of interpretation, and in 4% to poor performance of radiological images [61]. In 10% of cases, they are due to unusual lesion characteristics, in 9% to errors in the systematisation of lesion detection and in 7% to the limited quality of mammography equipment [61]. Factors such as inattention, fatigue and lack of experience are also important [61]. Studies carried out in Maryland in the USA and in the Netherlands have shown that there is considerable inter- and intra-observer variability in the use of the BIRADS lexicon for interpreting mammograms [10,75]. In view of the central role played by radiological examinations in the diagnosis of breast cancer, only doctors with specific training in breast imaging should be authorised to carry out and interpret breast imaging, the double reading system should be introduced and only homologous equipment should be authorised in Burkina Faso. With the local availability of training courses for radiodiagnostic and medical imaging specialists, we have more and more radiologists. This is a major advantage for the introduction of dual reading. The BIRADS initiated by the ACR has been adopted by most countries and greatly facilitates the management of breast cancer [14,32,65,75]. However, its optimal application requires specific training of the radiologist in breast imaging [14]. As in developed countries, an accreditation system for breast imaging and quality assurance of mammography and ultrasound should be introduced.

4.9.Assessment of extension

Breast cancer is a locoregional and general disease. These characteristics mean that extension must be assessed before any treatment is started. According to the March 2016 version of the referential of the Assistance Publique des Hopitaux de Paris (AP HP) [65], the 03 options for the extension work-up are: - chest X-ray combined with abdominal ultrasound and bone scintigraphy; - thoraco-abdominopelvic CT scan combined with bone scintigraphy; - FDG PET scan.

In the context of our work, scintigraphy is not commonly performed; only 16 patients (3.19%) underwent scintigraphy, and PET scans are not available. None of these three options, the combined chest X-ray, abdominal ultrasound and scintigraphy, were performed by any of the patients, and for the 2^{e} option, the combined thoracoabdominopelvic scan combined with scintigraphy, only 16 patients (3.19%) had it. However, we found that 388 patients (77.29%) underwent a thoracic-abdominopelvic scan, abdominal ultrasound represented 277 patients (55.18%) and thoracic radiography 256 patients (51%). This explains why scintigraphy is not commonly performed in our practice. The thoraco-abdomino-pelvic CT scan was the most commonly performed examination in our study, at 77.29%, which was much higher than the results of koama et al, who found a rate of less than 30%[43]. Our study showed that patients with higher levels of education and socio-economic status were more likely to have undergone this examination. The combination of abdominopelvic ultrasound and thoracic radiography was performed in more than half of our cases. The extension work-up depends on the stage of the tumour and is not systematic. It is not necessary in the case of T1N0 and T1N1 tumours; it is discussed in the case of T2N0 and T2N1 tumours and would depend on the clinical point of interest [65]. It should also be noted that some of the patients in whom extension work-up was requested were unable to undergo it for lack of financial resources. Our patients were metastatic in 38.05% of cases. This is a high rate and shows the need to make women more aware of the need for early consultation.

CONCLUSION

Imaging plays an important role in the management of breast cancer in our context. Mammography is the reference imaging technique for the early detection of breast cancer in the general population. It is frequently combined with breast ultrasound for complementary exploration of breast lesions. Breast cancer is a local and general disease. These characteristics mean that extension must be assessed before any treatment is started. Since PET scans are not available in Burkina Faso, scintigraphy is not widely used, and thoraco-abdominal-pelvic scans are difficult to perform in some low-income patients, which limits clinicians in prescribing an initial conventional extension assessment, which remains the key to initiating appropriate treatment. Breast cancer is a real public health problem worldwide and in Burkina Faso. It is therefore important to take action to reduce the morbidity and mortality rates associated with this disease.

SUGGESTIONS

To the Minister for Health and Public Hygiene

- Accelerate the implementation of the 2021 strategic cancer plan 2025;
- Encouraging multidisciplinary consultation meetings;
- Making universal health insurance operational;
- Subsidising chemotherapy;
- Make the existing cancer centres in Ouagadougou and Bobo-Dioulasso operational;
- Strengthen the technical resources of the imaging and radiodiagnostic departments of university hospitals to optimise extension assessments;
- Making PET scanners available in university teaching hospitals in Burkina Faso;

To learned societies

- To provide training workshops in the form of post-graduate courses (EPU) on breast cancer imaging in general and on the initial extension assessment and follow-up of breast cancer in particular;

To the Directors General of the University Hospitals and the Schiphra Protestant Hospital

- Electronic patient records;
- Enhancing the skills of radiologists in biological imaging;

To patients

- Regular breast cancer screening;
- Consult us if you notice the slightest abnormality or if you have any doubts;

REFERENCES

1. **Aka E, Horo A, Koffi A, Fanny M, Didi-Kouko C, Nda G, et al.** Single-centre African experience of personalised breast cancer management in Abidjan: challenges and prospects. Gynecol Obstet Fertil Senol. 2021;49(9):684- 90.
2. **Alkabban FM, Ferguson T. Breast cancer.** In: StatPearls [Online]. Treasure Island (FL): StatPearls Publishing; 2022 [accessed 2022 Mar 3]. Available from: http://www.ncbi.nlm.nih.gov/books/NBK482286/
3. **ANGLADE, E.** Les biopsies mammaires : indications et criteres de qualite. Journal de Radiologie, 2005, vol. 86, no 10, p. 1398.
4. **Anne Tardivon.** Imagerie de la femme, senologie ; Editions Lavoisier, Annee 2015, P.545.
5. **Anwar SL, Raharjo CA, Herviastuti R, Dwianingsih EK, Setyoheriyanto D, Avanti WS, et al.** Pathological profiles and clinical management challenges of breast cancer emerging in young women in Indonesia: a hospital-based study. BMC Women Health. 2019;19(1):1-28.
6. **Ataollahi M, Sharifi J, Paknahad M, Paknahad A.** Breast cancer and associated factors: a review. J Med Life. 2015;8(4):6- 11.
7. **Ba DM, Ssentongo P, Agbese E, Yang Y, Cisse R, Diakite B, Traore CB, Kamate B, Kassogue Y, Dolo G, Dembele E, Diallo H, Maiga M.** Prevalence and determinants of breast cancer screening in four sub-Saharan African countries: a population-based study. BMJ Open. 1 Oct 2020;10(10):e039464.
8. **Bakkach J, Mansouri M, Derkaoui T, Loudiyi A, Fihri M, Hassani S, et al.** Clinicopathologic and prognostic features of breast cancer in young women: a series from North of Morocco. BMC Women Health. 2017;17(1):1-106.
9. **Bambara HA, Zoure AA, Sawadogo AY, Ouattara AK, Ouedraogo NLM, Traore SS, Bakri Y, Simpore J**. Breast cancer: descriptive profile of 80 women attending breast cancer care in the Department, Pan Afr Med J 2017.
10. **Berg WA, Campassi C, Langenberg P, Mary J. Sexton.** Breast Imaging Reporting and Data System Inter- and Intraobserver Variability in Feature Analysis and Final Assessment. American Journal of Roentgenology. 2000;174: 1769-1777. Doi: 10.2214/ajr.174.6.1741769
11. **Boxshall M, Kiendrebeogo JA, Kafando Y, Tapsoba C, Straubinger S, Metangmo PM.** Presentation of the Free Health Care Policy in Burkina Faso. Washington DC: Health and Development Research and ThinkWell; 2020 p. 1-75
12. **Brunotte F, Berriolo-Riedinger A, Cochet A, Toubeau M, Dygai-Cochet I, Riedinger JM**. Place de l'imagerie dans revaluation de l'efficacite des traitements dans le cancer du sein. Medecine Nucl. 2010;34(1):58-65.

13. **Burnside ES, Sickles EA, Bassett LW et al.** The ACR BI-RADS Experience: Learning From History J Am Coll Radiol. 2009 Dec; 6(12): 851-860. doi: 10.1016/j.jacr.2009.07.023

14. **Cambier L.** Comment j'interprete une mammographie de depistage (mammotest). J Radiol 2002, 81 ;521- 528.

15. **Cheng S-A, Liang L-Z, Liang Q-L, Huang Z-Y, Peng X-X, Hong X-C, et al.** Breast cancer laterality and molecular subtype likely share a common risk factor. Cancer Manag Research. Dove Press; 2018;10:6549- 54.

16. **Cohen-Haguenauer O.** Hereditary predisposition to breast cancer. Med Sci. 2019;35(2):138- 51.

17. **Council of Ministers.** Decree n°2016-311-PRES/PM/MS/MATDSI/MINEFID of 29 April 2016 on free care for women and children under five living in Burkina Faso. BFA-2016-R-104122 29 Apr 2016 p. 1- 2.

18. **Dabakuyo-Yonli S, Arveux P.** Epidemiology of breast cancer. Rev Prat. 2020;70(7):726- 9.

19. **Delma S.** Apport de la chimiotherapie dans la prise en charge des cancers du sein dans trois structures sanitaires publiques de la ville de Ouagadougou, Burkina Faso: a propos de 65 cas. These de Doctorat d'etat en medecine, université de Ouagadougou BURKINA FASO. 2011; p. 146.

20. **Dem A, Traore B, Dieng MM, Diop PS, Ouajdi T, Lalami MT, Diop M, Dangou JM, Toure P.** Les cancers gynecologiques et mammaires a l'Institut du cancer de Dakar. Cah Detudes Rech Francoph Sante. 2 Sept 2008;18(1):25-9.

21. **Doudouh A, Biyi A, Oufroukhi Y, Zekri A**. Place de la scintigraphie osseuse au MDP-Tc99m dans le bilan d'extension initiale du cancer du sein (etude d'une serie de 102 malades). Medecine Nucl. 2008;32(11):585-8.

22. **Dujoncquoy S, Migeot V, Gohin-Perio B. Dujoncquoy S, Migeot V, Gohin-Perio B.** Information sur le depistage organisé du cancer du sein: etude qualitative aupres des femmes et des medecins en Poitou-Charentes. Sante Publique 2006; 4(18) :533-47.

23. **Engbang JPN, Essome H, Koh VM, Simo G, Essam JDS, Mouelle AS, Essame JLO.** Breast cancer in Cameroon, histo-epidemiological profile: about 3044 cases. Pan Afr Med J [Internet]. 2015 [cited 12 Oct 2023];21(1). Available from: https://www.ajol.info/index.php/pamj/article/view/132963

24. **Eric Barthelme** histoire de la notion du cancer Histoire des Sciences medicales 15, 167-172, 1981.

25. **Espina C, McKenzie F, dos-Santos-Silva** I. Delayed presentation and diagnosis of breast cancer in African women: a systematic review. Annals of Epidemiology. 2017;27(10):659- 71

26. Fouhi ME, Benider A, Gaëtan KZA, Mesfioui A. Epidemiological and anatomopathological profile of breast cancer at CHU Ibn Rochd, Casablanca. Pan Afr Med J. 9 Sep 2020; 37:41.

27. Gehlert S, Hudson D, Sacks T. A critical theoretical approach to cancer disparities: breast cancer and the social determinants of health. Front Public Health. 2021;9:674736.

28. Guindo F. Breast cancer in women under 40 in Mali: epidemiological, histopathological and immunohistochemical aspects. [Internet] [Thesis]. Universite des Sciences, des Techniques et des Technologies de Bamako; 2022 [cite 13 Oct 2023]. Available from: https://www.bibliosante.ml/handle/123456789/5736

29. Haas BM, Kalra V, Geisel J, et al. Comparison of tomosynthesis plus digital mammography and digital mammography alone for breast cancer screening. Radiology. 2013;269(3):694-700.

30. Haute Autorite de Sante (HAS): breast cancer screening and prevention. February 2015. https://www.hassante.fr/portail/jcms/c_2024559/fr/depist age-et-prevention-du-cancer-du-sein

31. Hicks DG, Lester SC. Invasive ductal carcinoma (adenocarcinomas of no special type). In: Hicks DG, Lester SC, editors. Diagnostic pathology: breast . 2nd ed. Philadelphia : Elsevier; 2016. p. 238- 47

32. Hirko KA, Rocque G, Reasor E, Taye A, Daly A, Cutress RI, et al. The impact of race and ethnicity in breast cancer-disparities and implications for precision oncology. BMC Medicine. 2022;20(1):1-72.

33. Ibrahim NY, Sroor MY, Darwish DO. Impact of bilateral breast cancer on prognosis: synchronous versus metachronous tumors. Asian Pac J Cancer Prev. 2015;16(3):1007- 10.

34. Institut national de la statistique et de la demographie du Burkina Faso (INSD). Annuaire statistique 2020, November 2021, 362 pages.

35. Institut national du cancer. Breast cancer risk factors. www.e- cancer.fr, consulted on 01/09/2023

36. Kamga J, Moifo B, Sando Z, Guegang Goudjou E, Nko'o Amvene S, Gonsu Fotsin J. Reliability of users of the BI-RADS classification in a tropical environment for the prediction of malignancy of breast lesions , year 2013, p. 439 -444.

37. Kemfang. N. D, Ebune J.L, Ngassam A, Atangana J, Kabeyene A, Kasia J.M. Clinicohistopathological features and molecular markers of breast cancer in a group of patients at the Yaounde General Hospital -Cameroon. J Afr Cancer Afr J Cancer. 1 Aug 2015;7(3):108-12.

38. Kiendrebeogo IT, Zoure AA, Sorgho PA, Yonli AT, Djigma FW,

Ouattara AK, Sombie HK, Tovo SF, Yelemkoure ET, Bambara AH, Sawadogo AY, Bakri Y, Simpore J. Glutathione S-transferase M1 (GSTM1) and T1 (GSTT1) variants and breast cancer risk in Burkina Faso. Biomol Concepts. 1 Jan 2019;10(1):175-83.

39. **Kirkpatrick DR, Markov NP, Fox JP, Tuttle RM.** Initial surgical treatment for breast cancer and the distance traveled for care. Am Surg. 2021;87(8):1280- 6.

40. **KOAMA A, Ouedraogo P.A, DAO BEN A, OUEDRAOGO N.A.N, TIEMTORE KAMBOU B M A, ZONGO N**. Apport de la radiologie dans la prise en charge diagnostique et therapeutique des cancers du sein en milieu Burkinabe a propos de 219 cas, annale de l'universite Joseph Ki ZERBO _ serie D , vol 024, Juillet 2020.

41. **LAHLAIDI. A** Topographical anatomy - Anatomical and surgical applications, volume III Ibn Sina book, 1986, p. 1 -315.

42. **Larra F.** Manuel de cancerologie. Doin editeur Paris 1984; 239p

43. **LEFRANC J.P.** History of breast cancer treatments. Service de chirurgie gynecologique. 1st edition 1986: p57-61.

44. **Les cancers du sein chez la femme de moins de 40 ans dans la ville de Ouagadougou** : Aspects epidemiologies, cliniques et therapeutiques, a propos de 40 cas. [These de doctorat de medecine]. Ouagadougou: Universite Pr Joseph KI Zerbo; 2011, thesis n°218.

45. **Lotersztajn N, Hequet D, Mosbah R, Rouzier R.** Place du traitement chirurgical locoregional chez les patients présentant un cancer du sein metastatique d'emblee. Gynecologie Obstetrique Fertil. 1 Apr 2015;43(4):304-8.

46. **Ly M, Antoine M, Andre F, Callard P, Bernaudin JF, Diallo DA**. Le cancer du sein chez la femme de l'Afrique subsaharienne: etat actuel des connaissances. Bull Cancer (Paris). 2011;98(7):797-806.

47. **Majeed W, Aslam B, Javed I, Khaliq T, Muhammad F, Ali A, et al.** Breast cancer: major risk factors and recent developments in treatment. Asian Pac J Cancer Prev. 2014;15(8):3353- 8.

48. **Ministry of Health of Burkina Faso.** Annuaire statistique 2020 , April 2021,148pages.

49. **Ministry of Health**. Comprehensive health profile of Burkina Faso. Burkina Faso: WHO; 2017 p. 1- 50.

50. **Ministry of Health**. Rapport de l'enquete nationale sur la prevalence des principaux facteurs de risques communs aux maladies non transmissibles au Burkina Faso : enquete Steps 2013. Burkina Faso : WHO ECOWAS; 2014 p. 1-81.

51. **N'de Ouedraogo NA, Napon M, Kambou Tiemtore BMA et al.** Breast

nodules with benign radiological appearance in Ouagadougou (Burkina Faso): microbiopsy or monitoring? Breast nodules with benign radiological appearance in Ouagadougou (Burkina Faso): microbiopsy or monitoring? J Afr Imag Med 2018; 10(2):

52. N'Koua-M'Bon J-B, Bambara AT, Moukassa D, Gombe-Mbalawa C. Clinical and evolutionary characteristics of inflammatory breast cancer in Brazzaville. Bull Cancer (Paris). 1 Feb 2013;100(2):147-53

53. NETTER.F.H, KAMINA.P Atlas of human anatomy. 4 eme edition-Masson ;annee 2009 p.1- 552.

54. NIZARDJ Cancerologie gynecologie obstetrique. www.laconferencehippocrate.com, consulted on 06 September 2023

55. World Health Organization . Framework for implementing the global breast cancer initiative: assessing, strengthening and scaling up early detection and management of breast cancer: a policy brief. 2023;

56. World Health Organization (WHO). Frequency and cause of errors in cancer diagnosis. October 2005.http:/ /www.interscience.wiley.co m/cancer-. Accessed 04 April 2018.

57. World Health Organization. Framework for implementing the global breast cancer initiative: assessing, strengthening and scaling up early detection and management of breast cancer: a policy brief. 2023.

58. Palazzetti V, Guidi F, Ottaviani L, et al. Analysis of mammographic diagnostic errors in breast clinic. Radiol Med. 2016; 121(11):828-833.

59. Pierre Kamina anatomie climique tome III 3[e] edition maloine 27, rue l ecole de medecine -75006 Paris, 2009.

60. PONS.J. Y Abrege de senologie - Edition Masson Paris 1985. P.1 -165.

61. United Nations Development Programme. Human Development Report 2019 - beyond incomes, averages and the present: human development inequalities in the twenty-first century. New York: UNDP; 2019 pp. 1- 410.

62. AP-HP guidelines. Cancer du sein. March 2016. P.1 -36.

63. Sidibe Y. Survival of women with breast cancer in Mali: analysis of a cohort of 124 cases managed at the Centre Hospitalo-Universitaire du Point-G from January 2007 to October 2010. 2015 [cite 12 oct 2023]; Malian journal of science and technology 66-79, 2019.

64. Sinnadurai S, Kwong A, Hartman M, Tan EY, Bhoo-Pathy NT, Dahlui M, et al. Breast-conserving surgery versus mastectomy in young women with breast cancer in Asian settings. BJS Open. 2019;3(1):48- 55. nt of General and Digestive Surgery of CHU-YO. Pan Afr Med J. 26 Dec 2017;28:314.

65. Some.O.R, Bague.A.H, Konkobo.D, Hien D, Dembele A, Belemlilga.G.L.H, Konsegre.V et Zongo.N. Le Cancer du Sein a Bobo-

Dioulasso, Burkina Faso : Resultats de la Prise en Charge. Tech Sci Press. 4 Jan 2022;

66. SOUDRE. Profil des marqueurs tumoraux circulants CA 15-3 et ACE au cours de la chimiotherapie du cancer du sein a Ouagadougou (Burkina Faso). [Ouagadougou]: UNIVERSITE Joseph KI-ZERBO; 2020.

67. Stapleton SM, Oseni TO, Bababekov YJ, Hung Y-C, Chang DC. Race/ethnicity and age distribution of breast cancer diagnosis in the united states. JAMA Surgery. 2018;153(6):594- 5.

68. Sun Y-S, Zhao Z, Yang Z-N, Xu F, Lu H-J, Zhu Z-Y, et al. Risk factors and preventions of breast cancer. Int J Biol Sci. 2017;13(11):1387- 97.

69. Sung H, Ferlay J, Siegel RL, Laversanne M, Soerjomataram I, Jemal A, et al. Global cancer statistics 2020: GLOBOCAN estimates of incidence and mortality worldwide for 36 cancers in 185 countries. CA Cancer J Clin. 2021;71(3):209-49.

70. Taourel P. MRI assessment of diagnostic breast cancer: Journal Radiologique. 87(10):1222,2006.

71. THOMASSIN-PIANA J, JALAGUIER-COUDRAY Aurelie, COHEN Monique, et al. Lesions histologiques mammaires a risque: clasRsification actuelle et prise en charge. Imagerie de la Femme, 2017, vol. 27, no 2, p. 138-142.

72. Timmers JMH, Van DoorneNagtegaal HJ, Zonderland HM et al. The Breast Imaging Reporting and Data System (BI-RADS) in the Dutch breast cancer screening programme: its roleas an assessment and stratification tool. Eur Radiol (2012) 22:1717-1723DOI 10.1007/s00330-012-2409-2

73. Toure M, Nguessan E, Bambara AT, Kouassi YKK, Dia JML, Adoubi I. Factors related to late diagnosis of breast cancer in sub-Saharan Africa: the case of the Ivory Coast. Gynecologie Obstetrique Fertil. 1 Dec 2013;41(12):696-700.

74. Umoke IC, Garba ES. Breast cancer in North-Central Nigeria: challenges to good management outcome. Int Surg J. 2019;6(9):3105- 10.

75. V. Juhan, P. Siles, S.Coze, **Cancer du sein : sur diagnostic, sur traitement**, Fait-on trop de micro- ou de macro biopsies ? p 61-66.

76. Williams F, Thompson E. Disparities in breast cancer stage at diagnosis: importance of race, poverty, and age. J Health Dispar Res Pract. 2017;10(3):34-45.

77. Wilson J, Sule AA. Disparity in early detection of breast cancer. In: StatPearls [Online]. Treasure Island (FL): StatPearls Publishing; 2022 [accessed 2022 Mar 12]. Available from: http://www.ncbi.nlm.nih.gov/books/NBK564311/

78. WORLD HEALTH ORGANIZATION, et al. Global breast cancer initiative implementation framework: assessing, strengthening and scaling-up of services for the early detection and management of breast cancer. World Health Organization, 2023.

79. Zanga S, Napon M, OUATTARA B, Diallo O, Mare V, BAMOUNI Y, et al. Mammographic screening and diagnostic difficulties of breast diseases at Yalgado Ouedraogo teaching hospital (Chu-Yo) of Ouagadougou. Sci Sante. 2017;40(2).

80. Zeeneldin AA, Ramadan M, Elmashad N, Fakhr I, Diaa A, Mosaad E. Breast cancer laterality among Egyptian patients and its association with treatments and survival. J Egypt Natl Canc Inst. 2013;25(4):199- 207.

81. Zongo N, Millogo-Traore FDT, Bagre SC, Bague AH, Ouangre E, Zida M, et al. Place de la chirurgie dans la prise en charge des cancers du sein chez la femme au centre hospitalier universitaire Yalagdo Ouedraogo: A propos de 81 cas. Pan Afr Med J 2015; 22: 117. Pan Afr Med J. 2015;22:117.

ICONOGRAPHY

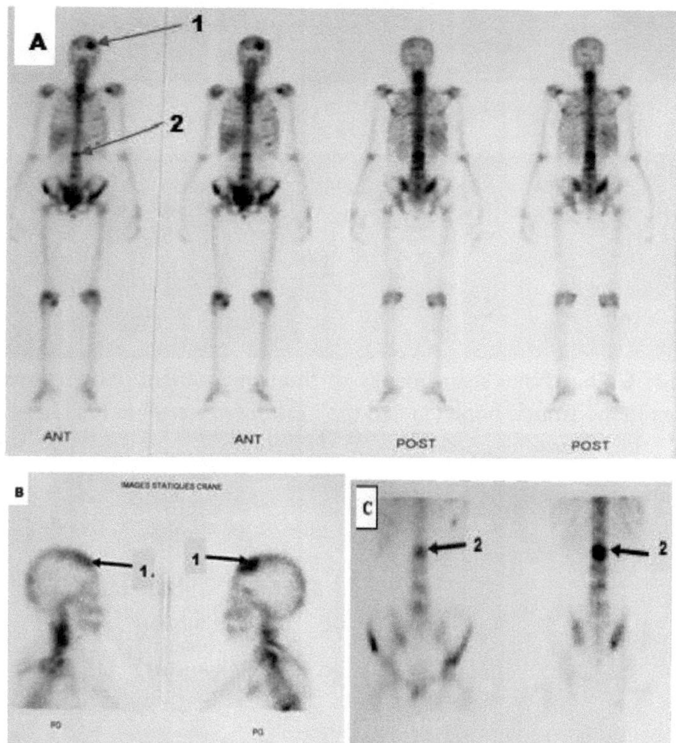

Figure 11: Technetium-99 (99mTch) bone scan of a 45-year-old woman with breast cancer as part of her initial extension work-up showing bone metastases in the skull **(1)** and lumbar spine at L2 **(2)**.

Source: Nuclear Medicine Department CHU-Yalgado OUEDRAOGO **A:** Overall view of the entire skeleton; **B:** Skull skeleton **C:** Spine skeleton; **1:** Hyperfixation of radiotracer in the frontal bone in relation to the metastasis; **2:** Hyperfixation of radiotracer in the lumbar vertebra L2 in relation to the metastasis.

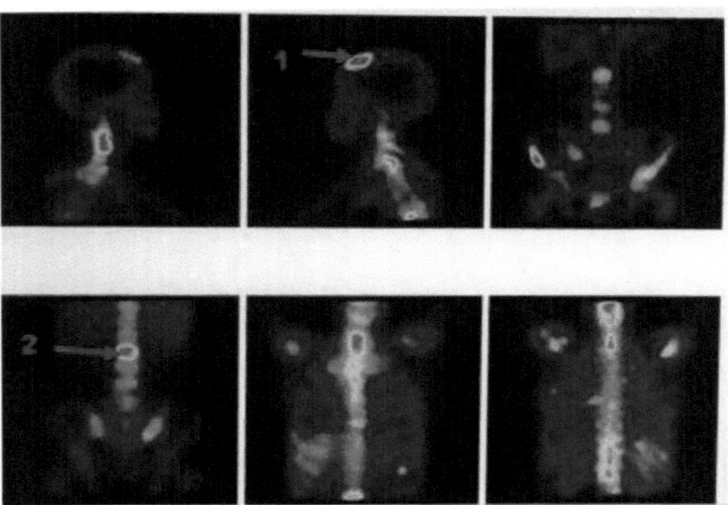

Figure 12: Colour bone scan images of the same patient above showing bone metastases in the frontal bone (1) and the L2 lumbar vertebra (2).

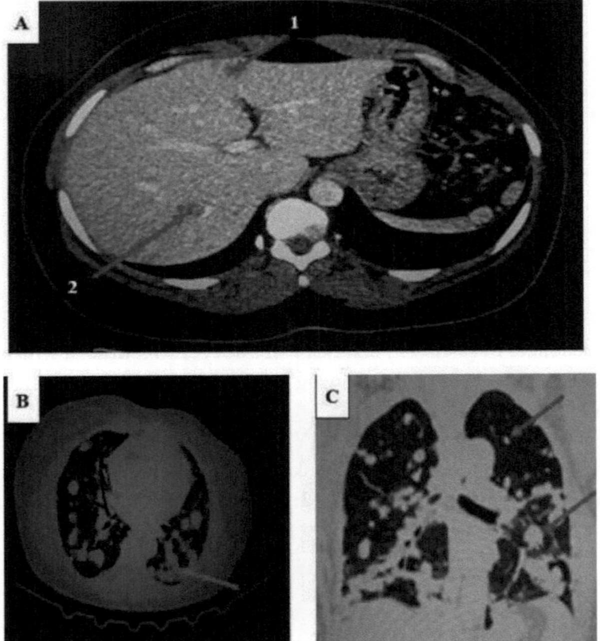

Figure 13: Thoraco-abdomino-pelvic CT scan of a woman with breast cancer as part of her initial extension work-up, showing hepatic (A) and pulmonary (B and C) metastases.

A: Axial section through the liver at portal time showing hypodense nodules in segments IV **(1)** and VII **(2)** associated with hepatic metastases.
B and C: Axial section through the thorax (B) in a parenchymal window with coronal reformation (C) showing multiple pulmonary nodules of varying size (red arrows) giving a "balloon laceration" image in relation to pulmonary metastases.

APPENDICES

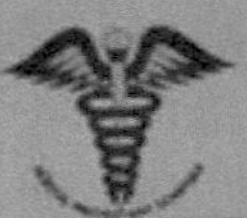

HÔPITAL PROTESTANT SCHIPHRA

BURKINA FASO
Unité-Progrès-Justice

MINISTERE DE LA SANTE
ET DE L'HYGIENE PUBLIQUE
Région du Centre
Direction Régionale de la Santé du Centre
District [illegible] de Nongr'Massom
HÔPITAL PROTESTANT SCHIPHRA

Ouagadougou le,10 Novembre 2023

Au

PrAg.KAMBOU-TIEMTORE
Bénilde Marie Ange
Ouagadougou

Objet : [illegible] demande d'Autorisation
de Collecte de données
[illegible] DAM 07112023/

Cher Professeur ;

[illegible] suite à votre lettre en date du 30 octobre 2023 sollicitant une autorisation de collecte [illegible] à l'*Hôpital Protestant SCHIPHRA* au profit de l'étudiant **KO Inéo Hamed** inscrit [illegible] de thèse de doctorat en médecine à l'Université ***Joseph KI- ZERBO*** et menant des [illegible] votre responsabilité, dont le thème est « **Bilan d'extension initial du cancer du sein à Ouagadougou**»; j'ai le plaisir de vous informer par la présente que je marque mon accord pour la réalisation de cette collecte.

[illegible] pourra prendre attache avec mes collaborateurs dans l'unité de gynéco-obstétrique pour les aspects pratiques de la collecte.

[illegible] en vous souhaitant une bonne réception de la présente, je vous adresse Cher Professeur l'expression de ma Franche Collaboration.

La Directrice Générale

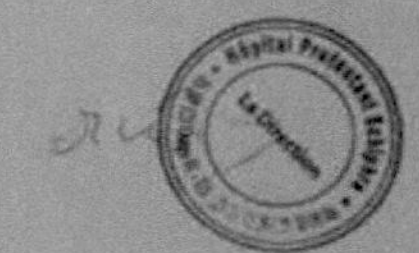

- Ampliation :
- *Chef de service de Gynéco-obstétrique*
- *[illegible] concerné*
- Archives

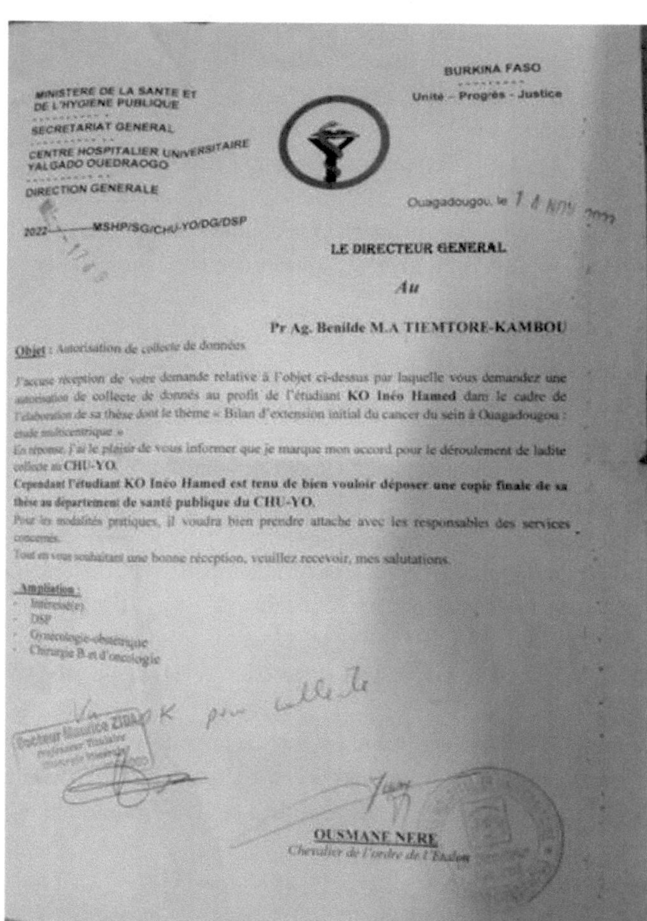

MINISTERE DE LA SANTE ET DE L'HYGIENE PUBLIQUE
SECRETARIAT GENERAL
CENTRE HOSPITALIER UNIVERSITAIRE YALGADO OUEDRAOGO
DIRECTION GENERALE

2022-_____MSHP/SG/CHU-YO/DG/DSP

BURKINA FASO
Unité – Progrès - Justice

Ouagadougou, le 14 NOV 2022

LE DIRECTEUR GENERAL

Au

Pr Ag. Benilde M.A TIEMTORE-KAMBOU

Objet : Autorisation de collecte de données

J'accuse réception de votre demande relative à l'objet ci-dessus par laquelle vous demandez une autorisation de collecte de donnés au profit de l'étudiant **KO Inéo Hamed** dans le cadre de l'élaboration de sa thèse dont le thème « Bilan d'extension initial du cancer du sein à Ouagadougou : étude multicentrique »

En réponse, j'ai le plaisir de vous informer que je marque mon accord pour le déroulement de ladite collecte au **CHU-YO.**

Cependant l'étudiant KO Inéo Hamed est tenu de bien vouloir déposer une copie finale de sa thèse au département de santé publique du CHU-YO.

Pour les modalités pratiques, il voudra bien prendre attache avec les responsables des services concernés.

Tout en vous souhaitant une bonne réception, veuillez recevoir, mes salutations.

Ampliation :

- Intéressé(e)
- DSP
- Gynécologie-obstétrique
- Chirurgie B et d'oncologie

Vu OK pour collecte

OUSMANE NERE
Chevalier de l'ordre de l'Etalon

Appendix 1: Collection form

Collection site:Collection date /.../....

I . **SOCIO-DEMOGRAPHIC DATA**

Last name: First name(s) :

AgeAns Sex : M / / F / / Residence : Urban / / Rural /
/

Level of education: no level / / primary / / secondary and university / /

Profession : Housewife / / employee / / entrepreneur / / shopkeeper / / farmer / / unemployed / / other profession / /

II **CLINICAL DATA**

History: family history of breast cancer/ / family history of ovarian cancer/ / personal history of breast cancer/ / personal history of ovarian cancer / / Oral contraception / /

Gestite : PariteMenopause / / Age of menarche

Circumstances of discovery :

Individual screening // Screening campaign // Nodule or mass breast / / inflammatory breast / / axillary adenopathy / / distant metastasis/ / other circumstances / / specify other circumstances

Clinical signs :

General status: WHO stage I / / WHO stage II / / WHO stage III / / WHO stage IV / /

Location of tumour: left breast/ / right breast/ / bilateral/ /

Nodule or breast mass / / Inflammatory breast / / Axillary adenopathy / / Respiratory sign / / Spinal pain / / Neurological sign / / Abdominal sign / / Other sign / / specify other sign

III **PARACLINICAL DATA**

Diagnostic imaging: breast ultrasound // echo-mammography/ / mammography/ /

Tumour size 1:.. mm Tumour size 2: Mm

ACR classification: ACR 2/ / ACR 3/ / ACR 4/ / ACR 5/ /.

Pre-therapeutic anatomopathology :

Histological type: Nonspecific infiltrating carcinoma (NSC) / / Invasive lobular carcinoma (ILC) / / / / Invasive lobular carcinoma (ILC) / / / NSC)

Mucinous carcinoma // Other histological type // Specify other type

- ----------- - -------- - - - - ----------- - -------- - - - - ----------- - -------- - - - ------

Scarff Bloom and Richardson histoprognostic grade: Grade I / / Grade II / / Grade III //

Vascular emboli: yes/ /no/ /

Assessment of extension :

Axillary ultrasound // MRI of the breast // MRI of the breast // MRI of the breast // MRI of the breast

Thoracic-abdominal-pelvic CT scan // Chest CT scan // Thoracic CT scan // Thoracic CT scan // Thoracic CT scan // Thoracic CT scan // Thoracic CT scan

Abdominal-pelvic scan/ / Chest X-ray: Abdominal ultrasound/ / Bone scan / / PET scan / / Other : ------.

Cerebral scan / cerebral MRI //.

Results of extension assessment :

Local extension: skin damage // nipple damage/ / tumour

multifocal // Multicentric tumour/ / Bilateral tumour/ / Bilateral tumour/ / Multifocal tumour/ / Multifocal tumour/ / Multifocal tumour/ / Multifocal tumour

Node extension: Axillary adenopathy // Number of nodes :

Metastasis :

Thoracic metastases / /

Pulmonary nodule/ / Number of nodules: less than 3// more than 3 //

Pulmonary micronodule // Pleuresy //

Abdominal and pelvic metastases / /

Hepatic metastases // Number of nodules: less than 3// more than 3 //

Abdominopelvic adenopathy/ / Ovarian metastasis/ / Ascites/ / Other abdominopelvic lesions//////////////////////////////

Bone metastases / /

Spinal location/ / pelvic location/ / rib location/ / other location //

Cerebral metastasis // Specify type of cerebral metastasis :

TNM classification

Tumour: T1// T2/ / T3// T4//

Ganglion: N0/ N1/ N2/ N3/ /

Metastasis: M0// M1//

TNM conclusion :

IV **THERAPEUTIC DATA**

Surgery / /

Breast-conserving surgery // mastectomy/ / axillary curage/ /

Chemotherapy / /

Neoadjuvant chemotherapy // chemotherapy // chemotherapy

Radiotherapy / /

Hormonotherapy / /

Other therapy/ / specify other therapy

V **PNONOSTIC DATA**

Patient vivant/ / Patient decede //

Delay from diagnosis to collection if patient alive //

Deadline from diagnosis to death if patient is deceased //.

HIPPOCRATIC OATH

In the presence of the teachers of this school and my dear fellow students, I promise and swear to be faithful to the laws of honour and probity in the practice of medicine. I will give my free care to the needy and I will never demand a salary above my work. Admitted to the interior of houses, my eyes will not see what goes on there; my tongue will keep silent about the secrets entrusted to me and my status will not serve to corrupt morals or encourage crime. Respectful and grateful to my teachers, I will give back to their children the education I received from their fathers. May men esteem me if I remain faithful to my promises. May I be shamed and despised by my colleagues if I fail to do so.

SUMMARY

Title: Initial extension assessment of breast cancer in Ouagadougou Multicentre study from 1er January 2021 to 31 December 2023

Objective: To study the initial extension of breast cancer in Ouagadougou from 1er January 2021 to 31 December 2023.

Patients and method: This was a retrospective descriptive-analytical study covering a 3-year period from 1er January 2021 to 31 December 2023. We included in the study all patients with histologically confirmed breast cancer who had undergone an initial extension work-up and whose records included extension imaging studies.

Results: A total of 502 patients were included in the study, 494 of whom were women (98.41%) and 8 men (1.59%), with an average age of 48.53 years. A family history of breast cancer was found in 4.38% of patients. The tumours were non-specific infiltrating carcinomas (90.84%) and grade II SBRm in 69.32% of patients. Tumour involvement was predominant in the left breast (48.21%). Stage T3/T4 predominated, accounting for 85.06% of cases. 99% of patients had benefited from diagnostic imaging consisting of mammography and/or breast ultrasound; only the 5 cases of necrotic ulcerated tumours did not undergo diagnostic work-up**.** In our study, 93.62% of the cancers diagnosed were classified as BIRADS 4 or 5 on imaging. Tumours initially classified as BIRADS 3 (5.38%) turned out to be breast cancers. In the initial extension work-up, 77.29% of patients underwent a thoraco-abdomino-pelvic CT scan, 55.18% underwent abdominal ultrasound and 51% underwent a chest X-ray. Only 16 patients (3.19%) underwent scintigraphy, breast MRI was performed in 9 patients (1.79%) and PET scans are not available in Burkina Faso. There was a statistically significant association between the level of secondary or university education, salaried occupation and the performance of thoracoabdominopelvic scans.

Conclusion: Despite the improvement in the initial extension assessment by increasing the use of thoracic-abdominal-pelvic CT scans, much remains to be done, in particular to increase the use of bone scans, breast MRI and the availability of PET scans in Burkina Faso. This will enable us to meet international recommendations for optimising breast cancer management in Burkina Faso.

Key words : breast cancer, initial extension assessment

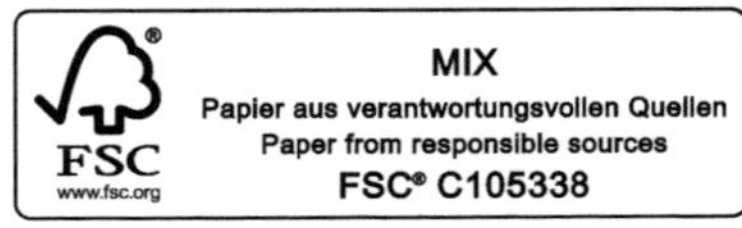

Printed by Books on Demand GmbH, Norderstedt / Germany